I0104890

JADED HEALTH

EVERY DAY HEALTH CHOICES
9 Simple Golden Rules for Living a Healthy Life

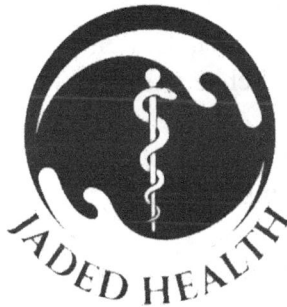

David Medansky

Copyright © 2024 by David Medansky

Jaded Health
Every Day Health Choices
9 Simple Golden Rules for Living a Healthy Life

All rights reserved. No part of this book may be reproduced or transmitted in any form or by any means, electronic or mechanical, including photocopying, recording, or by any information storage and retrieval system, without the written permission of the publisher or author, except as permitted by law. Manufactured in the United States of America, or in the United Kingdom when distributed elsewhere.

Paperback ISBN: 979-8-9905976-0-0
eBook ISBN: 979-8-9905976-2-4
Ingram Spark ISBN: 979-8-9905976-1-7
Library of Congress Control Number:2024915919
Front and Back Cover Design: 100 Covers
Interior design: Marigold 2K
Editing: Penny Hill, Michaela Gaffen Stone, and Karen Ketelaar
Contributing Author: Michaela Gaffen Stone

Published by Spotlight Publishing:
www.Spotlightpublishinghouse.com

Contact: www.JadedHealth.org

"If you fail to manage your own health and fitness, who will?"

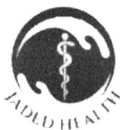

Waddell, AZ

DISCLAIMER

Before you implement or use any dietary, exercise, or health advice or suggestions from this book, please consult with a medical practitioner or qualified health professional.

All information provided in this book is intended for educational purposes only. Any health or dietary advice is not intended as a medical diagnosis or treatment. Statements contained in this book have not been evaluated by the Food and Drug Administration.

The author, publisher, and all other persons involved in producing this book deny all liability and loss in conjunction with the content provided herein, as well as any and all liability for any products or services mentioned or recommended in this book. The information contained herein is subject to personal research and the experiences of the author and has been recorded as accurately as possible at the time of publication. Due to changes and the availability of information provided to the public, you should not take any of the content as a source of reference without further research. The publisher and author are not responsible for any adverse effects or consequences resulting from the use of the suggestions, preparations, or procedures discussed in this book.

If you think you're suffering from any medical condition, then you should seek immediate medical attention. Results may vary. Causes for poor health vary from person to person. No individual results should be deemed as typical.

The information contained in this book is not intended as a substitute for consulting your physician or other healthcare provider. Any attempt to diagnose and treat an illness should be done under the direction of a healthcare professional.

MOTIVATE AND INSPIRE OTHERS!
"Share This Book"

This book is being given to:

_____

Because I care about you and your health,

From:

_____

*"Love yourself enough
to live a healthy life because time and
health are two precious assets we don't
appreciate until they are gone."*

—David Medansky
The Health Guy

MOTIVATE AND INSPIRE OTHERS!
"Share This Book"

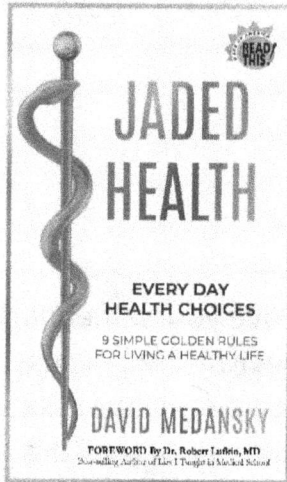

Retail Price $29.95
Special Quantity Discounts

5 – 20 Books	$19.95
21-99 Books	$17.95
100-499 Books	$13.95
500-999 Books	$ 9.95
1,000+ Books	$ 7.95

TO PLACE AN ORDER CONTACT
David Medansky, Inc.
18641 W. Alice Avenue
Waddell, Arizona 85355
(602) 721-5218
davidmedansky@gmail.com
www.JadedHealth.org

How to Effectively Bring
Jaded Health
Into Your Organization

1. **Keynote Presentation** (Ideal for Conferences, Conventions, & Retreats) Any organization that wants to develop their people to become "extraordinary" needs to hire David Medansky for keynote and/or workshop training!

2. **Jaded Health Training** (Ideal for in Office Events, Conferences, Conventions, & Retreats) facilitated by David Medansky, The Health Guy, is a three hour session aimed at teaching how to overcome challenges, have major breakthroughs, and achieve improved overall health. In this training, every participant will craft a personalized action plan capable of giving them more energy, better cognitive ability, and improve overall health. More importantly, it shows them how they can get started.

3. **Group Coaching** is facilitated by David Medansky, The Health Guy, this two hour session is aimed at alerting participants to the deceptive marketing tactics used by the food, drug, and weight-loss industries to manipulate them into purchasing their products that put the companies profits above the health of the participants. With this coaching, participants will receive tips, suggestions, and ideas to overcome the marketing tactics perpetrated by these companies.

TO CONTACT OR BOOK DAVID

David Medansky, Inc.
18641 W. Alice Avenue
Waddell, Arizona 85355
(602) 721-5218
davidmedansky@gmail.com
www.JadedHealth.org

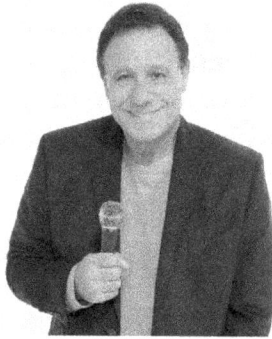

Dedication

This book is dedicated to you, the reader.

The Jaded Health Team is dedicated to informing, educating, and teaching individuals about making everyday healthy food choices and building healthy habits, as well as alerting you to the deceptive marketing tactics used by the food, pharmaceutical, and weight-loss industries, which prioritize their profits over your health. Our goal is to empower you to adopt a healthier lifestyle so you can enjoy life to the fullest.

About the Front Cover
Something You Might Not Know

The front cover of this book depicts the Staff of Asclepius, a single serpent wrapped around a long staff not to be confused with the Staff of Caduceus which shows a short staff with two serpents intertwined around it and two outstretched wings on the top.

The Staff of Asclepius is associated with healing and medicine whereas the Staff of Caduceus is identified with thieves, merchants, and messengers; an erroneous representation to symbolize a physician. In other words, the Staff of Caduceus is not the real symbol of medicine.

Nine Needs of the Body

Every person must have the following nine items to exist (survive) and thrive:

1. Air – Oxygen
2. Water – Pure water, not just liquids such as soda, diet soda, fruit juice, or fruit-flavored beverages.
3. Sleep – A minimum of 7 to 8 hours of quality sleep.
4. Food – Real whole food, not processed and manufactured foods.
5. Physical Movement – Physically active such as walking or stretching.

Note: The best way for you to lose unwanted body fat is by just simply walking. It doesn't have to be high intensity or uphill – just simply walk thirty minutes to an hour a day.

6. Sunlight
7. Non-energy Nutrients – Essential vitamins and minerals not produced by our bodies that you can only get through food.
8. Physical Touch and Community
9. Proper Elimination of Toxins

Your objective is to change your unhealthy eating habits into healthy ones. *To build a new lifestyle so that you can thrive instead of merely surviving*. A sailboat that changes course just one degree, over time will end up in a different place… and so will you. The best advice I can give you is to *be consistent* and give yourself plenty of *time*.

Don't quit. Just because you don't see results immediately, don't give up. You may not see changes, however, every smart choice you make is affecting you in ways you'd never imagine. It is the smallest, seemingly inconsequential changes done consistently over time that can make the biggest difference to successfully improving your health and living a healthy lifestyle.

A sailboat that changes course just one degree, over time will end up in a different place... and so will you. The best advice I can give you is to be consistent and give yourself plenty of time.

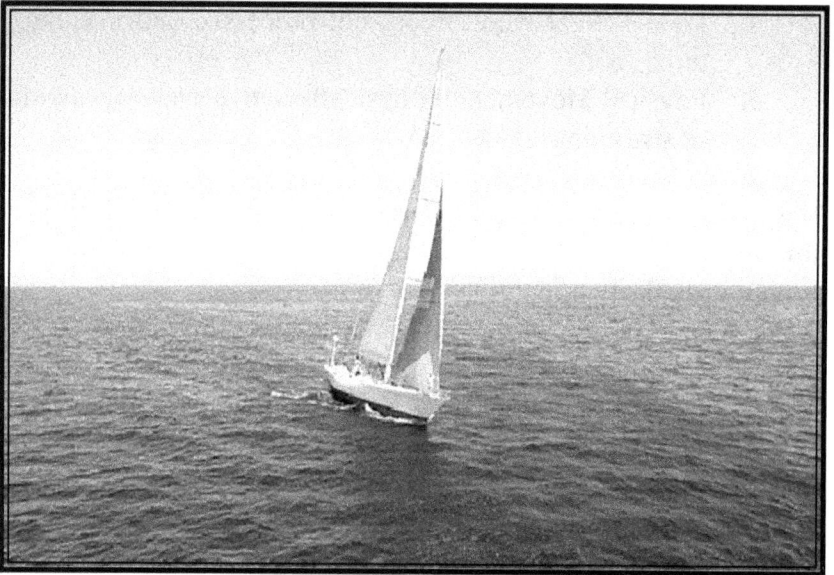

"Perfection is not attainable, but if we chase perfection, we can catch excellence."
— Vince Lombard

Contents

"Don't overlook the basics. Don't ignore the foundation. How long can a tree remain standing without the roots?"

– James Clear
Author of *Atomic Habits* and Keynote Speaker

Foreword

By Dr. Robert Lufkin, MD
Author of *Lies I Taught in Medical School*, full professor
at both the UCLA and USC Schools of Medicine

As a physician and a metabolic health and longevity expert, I've spent years navigating the complex landscape of modern medicine, striving to uphold the principles of integrity, empathy, and patient-centered care. Yet, in my journey, I've come to realize that the profession I once revered is not without its flaws. In fact, modern medicine is lying to you. In my book, *Lies I Taught in Medical School*, I expose the hypocrisy and inadequacies that permeate the medical establishment for the common underlying causes of most chronic diseases that have been overlooked for decades, challenging the status quo, and calling for a change in thinking in the way we approach health and wellness.

In the midst of this tumultuous landscape, David Medansky's ***Jaded Health Everyday Health Choices 9 Simple Golden Rules for Living a Healthy Life*** offers a much-needed beacon of hope and inspiration. Through a collection of parables and short stories, Medansky invites readers to embark on a transformative journey toward better health, free from the confines of conventional medical wisdom and outdated dogma.

In ***"Jaded Health,"*** Medansky skillfully weaves together timeless wisdom with practical insights, guiding readers on a path to reclaiming vitality and embracing a life of wellness. Through the lens of relatable characters facing familiar health challenges, Medansky invites us to reflect on our own lives and consider how we can apply these lessons to our own health journey.

One of the most compelling aspects of *"Jaded Health"* is its emphasis on simplicity and sustainability. In a world inundated with quick-fix solutions and fad diets, Medansky reminds us that true health is not about following the latest trends or adhering to rigid rules, but rather about cultivating habits that nourish our bodies, minds, and spirits for the long term.

As a physician who has witnessed firsthand the limitations of conventional medicine, I am heartened by Medansky's comprehensive approach to health and wellness. By prioritizing whole, nutrient-dense foods, fostering a positive mindset, and engaging in regular physical activity, Medansky provides readers with a roadmap for living a healthy life that transcends the confines of traditional medical thinking.

As you journey through the pages of "Jaded Health," I encourage you to approach it with an open mind and a willingness to challenge the status quo. Don't let the simplicity of the 9 Simple Golden Rules for Living a Healthy Life fool you. They are game changers. Embrace the wisdom contained within the stories and parables and let them serve as a catalyst for change in your own life. May you find inspiration, empowerment, and renewed vitality as you embark on your own journey toward better health.

— Dr. Robert Lufkin, MD,
Full professor at both the UCLA and USC Schools of Medicine. In addition to being a practicing physician, he is the author of more than 200 peer-reviewed scientific papers and 14 books that are available in six languages. Among his many inventions, including several patents in artificial intelligence, he developed an MR-compatible biopsy needle which is used worldwide today as the "Lufkin Needle." He is active on social media with more than 250,000 followers.

A Message to You!

9 Simple Golden Rules for Living a Healthy Life

Old: I'm dieting

New: "I'm Making Every Day Health Choices"

According to Merriam-Webster, the meaning of *Jaded* is fatigued by overwork: exhausted. Collins Dictionary defines Jaded as tired; worn-out; wearied. 2. Dulled, or satiated, as from overindulgence; a *jaded* appetite. And according to Oxford Languages, Jaded is defined as tired, bored, or lacking enthusiasm, typically after having had too much of something. Today, individuals, such as yourself, are tired and worn out because of the deception and manipulation of the food, pharmaceutical, diet and weight-loss industries. Michaela Gaffen Stone put it this way, "The food industry gets you sick, big pharma keeps you sick, and the diet and weight-loss industries are aiding and abetting both of them."

If you're ready to have more energy, feel better, look better, have enhanced mental clarity, and improve your overall health, then this book is for you.

"Every Day Health Choices" is defined as "simple everyday things that you can do and more importantly, will do." It is a process to successfully make healthier food choices and live a healthy lifestyle. It is a change in basic assumptions from the "diet" and weight-loss industries so you can have a healthy and active lifestyle. *"Every Day Health Choices"* means you want to be health-

ier. There are nine (9) Simple Golden Rules for Every Day Health Choices.

The information in this book will empower you to understand what is possible and how to do it. Imagine how you'll feel attending a high school class reunion, going to a special event such as a wedding and being told, "You look fabulous." Whether you are looking to increase your energy to keep up with your kids or grand kids and work obligations, lose weight, feel better, look better, or improve your health, this book is equipped with everything you need to get there and stay there – for life. Start your journey to a healthier new you!

Eating a healthy diet is about integrating small healthy habits that become second nature. It is these small seemingly inconsequential improvements done consistently and for an extended period of time that will make a big difference to your health in the long term. Think of it this way — a healthy diet is a long-term approach that keeps you in a healthier life, while a diet is a short-term solution that only works if the food restrictions are followed continuously.

You can never own your good health.
You can only rent it.
And the rent is due every day in the form
of the food and beverages you choose to eat and drink.
It comes down to the choices you make.

My mission in writing this book is to create a movement to expose the food, pharmaceutical, weight-loss, and diet industries, so you can stop wasting money on FAD (Fat and Desperate) diets that don't work and avoid being deceived by the marketing tactics used by the food companies that prioritize their profits over your health. You can elevate your own eating routines, behaviors, and habits so you too can improve your health, increase your vitality, and heighten your cognitive ability and mental alertness. And, without having to buy expensive meals, supplements, or products, and without needing to follow a specific exercise program. My goal is to make an impact by being an example and encouraging you and others who want to be healthier.

The magical ingredients necessary for your success to live a healthy lifestyle are given to you in this book. You just need to follow along. My wish for you is for you to enjoy your life to the fullest because when you eat for your health, everything else will take care of itself.

Throughout this book are short stories with life lessons. I've applied these teachings to eating healthier and living a healthy lifestyle in an effort to better communicate the messages and morals of these anecdotes as it might apply to your own life.

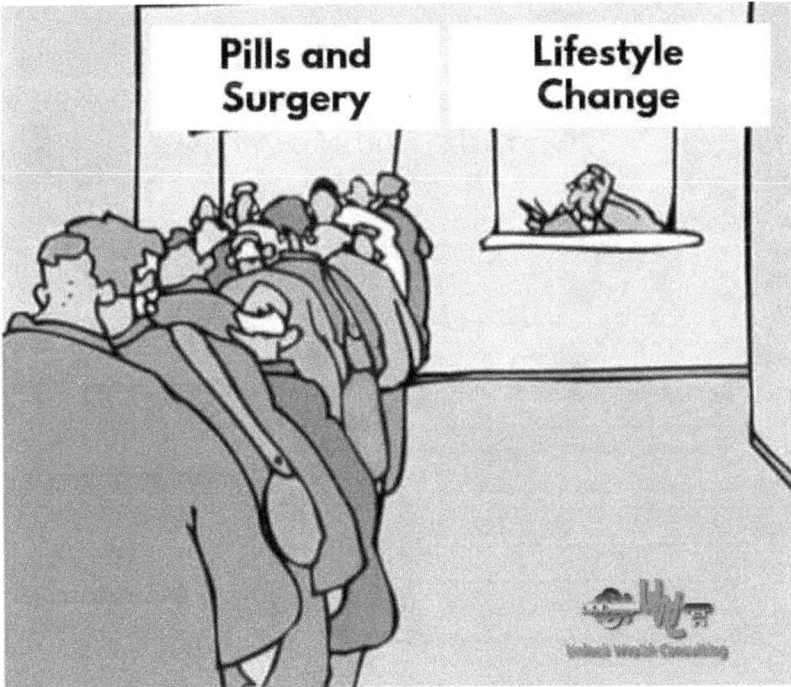

"An ounce of prevention is worth a pound of cure."

REMINDER

The reasons why I'm choosing to eat healthy:

1. That cute pair of shorts that don't fit me anymore

2. More energy

3. Better sleep quality

4. Overall feeing of wellbeing

5. Glowing skin / less acne

6. To get rid of my stomach problems

7. Healthier teeth and gums

8. Increased confidence

9. Decreased health risks

10. To enjoy life more

11. Because I care about myself and my body!!

Daily Prayer

Lord [Universe], thank you for blessing my efforts to make better food choices today.

Thank you for helping me to keep the vision of being healthier.

Thank you for watching over me as I seek to monitor all I eat and drink.

Thank you for helping me to enjoy food and to love and care for myself as I improve my health in a sustainable manner.

Lord [Universe], thank you for giving me energy as I walk more and become fit.

Thank you for guiding me as I strive to improve my health and blessing my efforts with sustainable improved health.

Thank you for helping me this day to make healthy choices and give me the strength to fight against destructive cravings that negatively affect my health.

Thank you for helping me to reject any unhealthy behaviors, routines, and habits that give me false comfort.

Thank you for giving me the grace to be strong and encouraging me to keep pushing forward.

Even though I am not at my ideal weight, I love, accept, and appreciate my body.

Amen.

A Dog Story

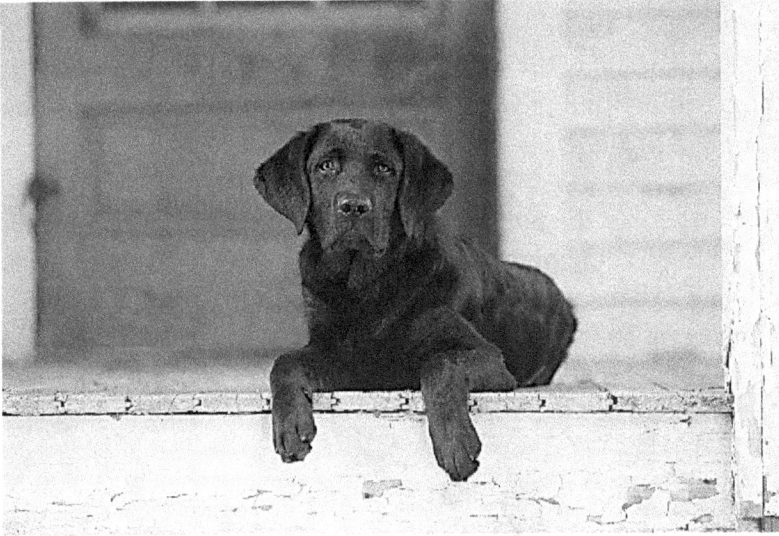

An old man and his three dogs are sitting on the porch. A neighbor is walking by and two of the dogs jump up and start to bark. The third dog, however, remains seated whimpering apparently in pain.

A few minutes later, the neighbor is returning home. Once again two of the dogs get up and start to bark. The third dogs still remained seated whimpering. The neighbor asks, "Is your dog that is whimpering okay?"

The old man responds, "No, he's not. He's sitting on a nail."

The confused neighbor looked bewildered. He asks the old man, "Why doesn't the dog just get up and move?"

The old man sipped his coffee and said, "Well, I guess it doesn't hurt bad enough for him to get up and move."

Are you the dog sitting on the nail being unhealthy? Are you tolerating being in poor shape and overweight?

Sometimes in life the pain we know is more comfortable than the pain we don't know. Especially because of the increased risk for Type 2 diabetes, heart attack, stroke, and other health issues that can be avoided and prevented with simple changes to your dietary intake and lifestyle.

A lot of people tolerate being unhealthy because it doesn't hurt enough to do something about it. Do you justify and make excuses for being exhausted and fatigued all the time? Are you frustrated having brain fog in the afternoon? What needs to happen for you to do something about it?

The Secret to Success

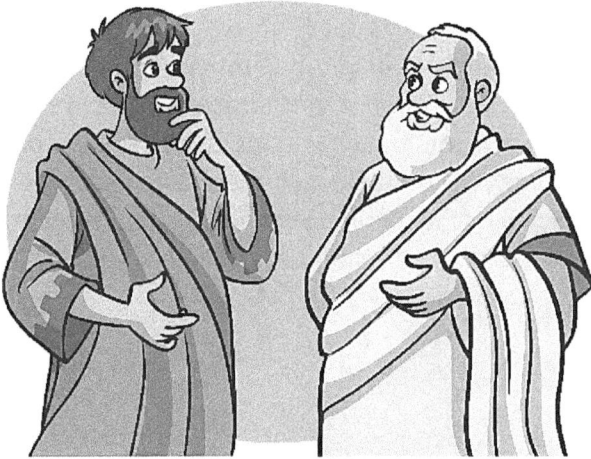

A young man asked Socrates, an ancient Greek philosopher, the secret of Success. Socrates told the young man to meet him near the river the next morning where he would be given the answer.

In the morning, Socrates and the boy met and began walking towards the river. They continued on into the river, past the point of the water covering their nose and mouth. At this time, Socrates dunked the boy's head into the water.

As the boy struggled, Socrates continued to push him deeper into the water. After a few seconds, Socrates pulled the boy's head up so he could get air. The boy gasped as he inhaled a deep breath of air.

Once the boy had an opportunity to catch his breath and regain his composure, Socrates asked, 'What were you fighting for when you were underwater?"

The boy answered, "Air!"

Socrates said, "There you have the secret to success. When you want to gain success as much as you wanted air when you were underwater, you will obtain it. That's the only secret."

The lesson of this story is that success starts with the desire to achieve something. If your motivation is weak, your results will be weak as well. Think about your desire to improve your health. How desperate are you to be healthier? Don't allow your environment or other people to influence the things that you genuinely want. Just because other people are comfortable being overweight, out of shape, and in poor health doesn't mean you need to be too.

Introduction

You've been lied to about eating healthy... and so was I.

Today, more than 150 million American adults are overweight. Loosely translated, that is more than 72 percent of the U.S. adult population. This means if you are at a social gathering with 10 friends, seven of you are overweight, of which four are clinically obese. Just look around.

How successful was your last diet? Probably not too good. Let's face it, diets tend to be extreme, temporary, hard to stick with, and potentially dangerous to your health.

Have you tried and failed at every diet and weight-loss program, including the big national brands? Conventional diets not only don't work, but they also make you miserable, and the word "diet" has "die" in it.

It is not your fault you did not lose weight on that diet. The diet is to blame. You did not fail the diet. The diet failed you because diets are designed to be unsuccessful.

More than 45 million Americans start a new diet each year. At any one time, more than 108 million Americans are on a diet. Yet, Americans are getting fatter. The biggest mistake you can make when attempting to lose weight is going on a diet. Some studies show that 95 percent of people fall short of their weight-loss goals on diets. The average person will attempt 4 to 5 new diets each year and 126 different diets during their lifetime.

How many diets have you attempted?

If you keep starting over, and over, and over, you'll never get anywhere.

The food, drug, and weight-loss industries are a racket to manipulate you to buy their products and services. Why would I say such a thing? Because Americans spend more than **$71 BILLION each year** on weight-loss products and services. And still, more than 72 percent of the U.S. population is overweight and unhealthy.

Plus, it is getting worse. In other words, if diets and weight loss programs worked, the diet and weight-loss companies would be out of business after a few years. We'd all be thinner and healthier.

Diets are about reaching a goal as opposed to lifestyle changes. This is one reason they fail. Because once many people reach their goal, they revert back to their old eating habits. Can you relate to this? Perhaps this is why you keep losing the same 10 pounds over and over again? Saying, "I'm on a diet" carries an inferred message that it is something you will eventually "go off of."

Another reason many popular diets go wrong is because they rely on you to have willpower, self-control, or discipline. For your health and weight-loss journey to succeed, you must find a way to remove all thinking, all discipline, and all willpower from the equation. If you need to rely on any of that, you are doomed. Many popular weight-loss programs are flawed because they primarily depend on continual willpower and self-control, or that you continue to buy their products and services. Instead, you want your eating habits and lifestyle to be enjoyable; a welcome second nature, rather than something that fills you with dread.

People love to believe they can lose weight on the latest trendy diet or magical supplement. I am here to tell you there are no shortcuts to being healthy and sustainable weight-loss.

There is no miraculous fruit, berry, nut, vegetable, or supplement to permanently lose weight. It does not exist. If there was, we'd all be thinner.

There is no lotion to rub on your belly to get rid of fat.

There is no genie in a bottle to grant your wish of being thinner and healthier.

In fact, you should never go on a diet. Instead, change your diet and your relationship with food. You must choose to make a conscious decision and act to improve your eating habits and lifestyle.

Now is the time to change your world as it relates to food. This means you must change your eating habits: when you eat, where you eat, how you eat, how much you eat, and what you eat.

Start now. Because if you put off until tomorrow what you can do today, and tomorrow never comes, you will never do what needs to be done. Mark Twain stated it best when he said, "Don't wait. The time will never be just right."

So why is it so difficult for you to eat healthy and live a healthy lifestyle? Most people fail because:

- It is difficult to get started.
- There is no magic formula.
- It is not a quick fix.
- It is challenging to sustain.
- There is no finish line.
- There is no one to hold you accountable.
- Even if you know what to do you might not know how to do it.
- And, with all the information available about healthy eating, dieting, and weight-loss, who or what do you believe to act upon?

Time to Act

Yesterday You Said Tomorrow

With respect to living a healthy lifestyle, there are three types of people: 1) those who think about being healthy yet do nothing, 2) those who talk endlessly about being healthy, yet do nothing, and 3) those who act to be healthy. Which one are you?

There is a saying, "The person who has great health, has a thousand dreams. The person who has bad health, has only one dream."

There is never a perfect or right time to begin living a healthy lifestyle because we all procrastinate and make excuses. Have you used as an excuse to justify delaying your health journey saying, "I'll start on Monday," "I'll start after the holidays," or "After our vacation?" You get the idea.

Ask yourself this, "If I delay and put off until tomorrow what I can start today, what might happen?" Here's a hint to your answer. If tomorrow never comes, it means if you keep putting off until tomorrow what you can start today, you will never start.

T. Harv Eker said, "One step in the right direction is worth 100 years of thinking about it." And, Lemony Snicket said, "If we wait until we're ready, we'll be waiting for the rest of our lives." However, legendary UCLA head basketball coach John Wooden said it best, "If you don't have the time to do it right, when will you have the time to do it over?"

Unfortunately, too many people wait until it's too late to decide to eat healthy and live a healthy lifestyle.

The Perception of Being Healthy Has Shifted

Americans Are Getting Fatter

Recently, a photo of people at the beach in the '70s was posted on Facebook. What is interesting about the photo was that few, if any, of the beachgoers are overweight.

In 1960, the average weight for men ages 20 to 74 was 166.3 pounds. The average waist size was 34 inches. In 2002 the average weight of a man dramatically increased to 191 pounds. In 2021, the average weight of a man was 197.9 pounds and their waist size expanded to 42 inches.

Meanwhile the average weight of a woman rose from 140.2 pounds in 1960 to 164.3 pounds in 2002 to 168.5 pounds in 2021. The average waist size of a female rose from 25 inches in the 60s to 39 inches in 2021.

Have you noticed a trend?

What will happen if you don't improve or change your eating habits?

Will you be like so many others and be diagnosed with Type 2 diabetes?

Will you suffer a stroke or heart attack?

Or will you end up in the hospital with some other debilitating disease or illness?

Worse yet, research shows that consuming certain foods high in sugar and artificial ingredients increases your risk for dementia and Alzheimer's disease.

Eating highly processed, ultra processed, and manufactured foods now causes more deaths than smoking.

Think about that. **Eating scientifically engineered (processed) foods now causes more deaths than smoking**. And seven out of every ten U.S. adults are overweight and four of those ten are clinically obese. Sobering statistics.

Researchers found that one in five (20 percent) of worldwide deaths is linked to unhealthy eating habits. What you eat, and don't eat, may pose a bigger threat to your health than smoking, drinking, and other common risk factors for premature death.

Research shows that 90 percent of heart attacks are preventable through dietary intake and physical activity. A Mediterranean type of diet combined with walking every day decreases mortality by 50 percent.

What is Your Motivation for Improved Health?

If I am unable to inspire you to start to improve your eating habits and live a healthy lifestyle, maybe I can use the fear of you being at higher risk for serious illness, infection, sickness, and possible death from your poor food choices and eating habits to motivate you.

Perhaps you are not concerned about yourself. If not, think of the impact a preventable food-related illness could have on your family, your business, loved ones, and others.

Les Brown said, *"The graveyard is the richest place on earth, because it is here that you will find all the hopes and dreams that were never fulfilled, the books that were never written, the songs that were never sung, the inventions that were never shared, the cures that were never discovered, all because someone was too afraid to take the first step, keep with the problem, or determined to carry out their dream."*

Imagine your hopes and dreams being cut short because you failed to take care of yourself by simply making better food choices and living a healthy life. It would be incredibly sad if you had a heart attack or stroke, or a chronic illness that prevented you from accomplishing your potential. All of these could have been avoided and prevented by making simple, easy-to-do, lifestyle changes.

So, what will scare you enough to change your eating habits to improve your health?

Perhaps you should talk to people with Type 2 diabetes, people who have suffered a stroke, a heart attack, or lost a foot or leg to diabetes. Better yet, talk to the loved ones who have lost parents, friends, relatives, and siblings way too early because of the poor food choices they made. Or have a conversation with someone who is taking care of a spouse or parent who has dementia.

Have you put off living a healthy lifestyle because it wasn't the perfect time, or you struggled with it? Each day, countless numbers of people say they will start eating healthier tomorrow. Unfortunately, for most of them, tomorrow never comes.

The reality is there is no perfect time to start living a healthy lifestyle. The best advice I can offer you is just start improving your eating habits and never stop. As Zig Ziglar so eloquently put it, "You don't have to be great to start, but you have to start to be great."

Nike had a message that really resonated with me: "Yesterday you said tomorrow." We all know that if we put off until tomorrow what we can do today, we are just kidding ourselves.

Waiting to do something until tomorrow is another fallacy. More excuses, more justification to delay, until it may be too late. Please don't delay implementing a process to improve and modify your eating behaviors. Act now! You'll either keep making excuses, have reasons, or you'll have results. Another Nike slogan is, "Just Do it." Perhaps it should be, "Just do it now!"

So, Who the Heck is David Medansky and Why Should You Listen to Me?

I am not a doctor. Nor am I a mental or health professional. However, I have been where you are. I understand the challenges, frustrations, and obstacles you will face along your journey to living a healthy lifestyle.

Maybe some of you are like me; we were fit and trim when we were younger. However, as with most people, life gets in the way, whether it be family or work obligations. Maybe you, like me, stopped exercising. Or, like me, you started eating more fast food and convenience foods. Instead of eating one scoop of ice cream, I'd eat an entire pint in one sitting. Or an entire canister of Pringles. If there was a special buy-one-get-one-free sandwich at a fast-food place, I'd eat both sandwiches. I was disgusted with myself. I couldn't believe my pants size ballooned up.

Perhaps, like me, the weight crept up on you.

Like many of you, I struggled with weight issues and dieting. I went on many different diets, looking for the perfect one. However, no matter what I did or what diet I attempted, I failed.

If I did lose weight, I wouldn't be able to keep it off.

Then something happened to turn my life around. I dubbed it my wake-up call. In July 2016, my doctor told me, based on my lab results and being significantly overweight, I had a 95 percent chance of a *fatal* heart attack. He gave me two options: 1) lose weight, or 2) find a new doctor because he did not want me to die on his watch. In most things, I am pleased to be in the 95th percentile, but not if it meant I was likely to die. Suddenly, my being significantly overweight was more than just embarrassing, it was lethal.

With that sword hanging over my head, I managed to shed 50 pounds over the next four months, nearly a quarter of my total body weight. More importantly, I have kept the weight off since then. Now I feel great, I have more energy, better mental clarity, and I have improved my overall health. That is what I want for you – for you to have more vitality, more energy, to feel better, look better, get rid of brain fog, and improve your overall health.

I learned how to lose weight without going on a diet, without exercising, without counting calories, and without needing to buy any special meals, supplements, or products. More importantly, I've kept the weight off. I did a tremendous amount of research on the subject. This much I know, when it comes to losing weight, keeping it off, and living a healthy life, not one size fits all.

In June of 2022, at age 67, I hiked Mt. Kilimanjaro.

Most people know what to do to eat heathier and live a healthier lifestyle. We just don't do it. Why? Why is it so difficult to live a healthy lifestyle? Probably because it's not what we can do, rather, it's what we will do. And that's the answer – knowing what you can do, yet not willing to do it.

Everyone Will Tell You How to Lose Weight, Few Will Tell You How to Become Healthy

After I released my unwanted and unhealthy weight, I started re-reading the health books I had read in the 1970s, such *as Sugar Blues* by William Dufty, books by Paul and Patricia Bragg, Jack LaLanne, Richard Simmons, and others to improve my eating habits and overall health.

Being a former lawyer, I am trained to do research. To sift through information and discern between fact, opinion, and fiction. While doing my research for healthy weight-loss, I was overwhelmed and inundated with the amount of information available. Thousands and thousands of books have been written about diet, nutrition, fitness, and exercise. Right now, there are more than 50,000 books available on Amazon pertaining to diet, weight-loss, health, fitness, and nutrition. At the grocery store checkout, you'll see hundreds of magazine articles written about health and wellness. Thousands of blogs and articles are available when you search Google and YouTube. Numerous weight-loss programs, both national and local, are advertised on TV, radio, and social media.

With all the information out there about health, wellness, and nutrition, who or what do you believe and act on? How do you choose? One expert will tell you one thing, another will say exactly the opposite. A third expert will then tell you the other two are both wrong.

As a lawyer, I spent my career seeing both sides of the fence – honest people and dishonest people. And when it comes to the food, pharmaceutical, and weight-loss industries, sadly, there are more dishonest people than there are those telling the truth. That's what makes living a healthy lifestyle so difficult.

Just like I had to read the fine print when I practiced law, I am now reading and exposing the fine print on food labels and diet programs. Now I want to unmask the food, pharmaceutical, diet, and weight-loss industries deceptive marketing tactics to help others to live a healthy lifestyle so you can reduce weight and keep it off, without going on a diet or dieting. Again, if weight-loss and diet programs worked, those companies would be out of business. They depend on repeat customers to stay relevant.

You will never improve your health until you change your daily eating habits and routines. The secret of you living a healthy lifestyle is found in your daily eating practices.

According to Cardiologist, Dr. Mimi Guarneri, "70 to 90 percent of chronic diseases is related to lifestyle and environment. Where you live, who you live with, what you eat, are you breathing clean air, are you drinking filtered clean water, what king of toxins are in your life, and so on."

Research also shows that 90 to 95 percent of your body weight and shape is determined by your diet, what you eat and drink, and only 5 to 10 percent is determined by your physical activity and other factors such as hormones or medical conditions. People always confuse exercising with weight-loss. You can shed weight without exercising.

However, you can never exercise enough to overcome poor eating habits.

Isn't that right Bob Harper of *The Biggest Loser* fame?

In early 2017, Bob Harper had a heart attack at the gym during his workout. He was only 52 years old. Being one of the biggest names in the fitness industry, Harper's heart attack came as a shock since many people believed he depicted excellent health.

After his heart attack, Harper made lifestyle changes to become healthier. He says, "I've been in the health and fitness industry for almost 30 years now, but I had to pivot my life and redefine the way that I ate and worked out." Now he primarily follows a Mediterranean diet.

Exercise is not the best way to lose weight. Exercising to lose weight is a myth. Here is why. Most people overestimate how many calories they burn during a workout and underestimate how many calories they consume. Plus, most people tend to eat more when they exercise because they're hungrier.

Fat and muscle weigh the same. Five pounds of fat weighs the same as five pounds of muscle. However, fat takes up more space than muscle. When you burn fat and increase muscle mass, you either won't lose weight or you will gain weight. Would this frustrate you if you put in the hours of exercising thinking you are losing weight only to see the scale read the same or more? For most people it becomes extremely discouraging, and then they quit.

Let me tell you about a client of mine, David Watson, who experienced this frustration. During one of our coaching and accountability telephone calls, David expressed his disappointment at not losing weight during the first few weeks of the program. He had modified his eating habits and lifestyle. However, the number on the scale remained the same.

In talking with David, he told me he had started walking about five miles each day, was riding his bicycle, and was exercising more. I asked him how his clothes fit. David replied that his clothes were loose. He also mentioned that other people were noticing that he looked slimmer.

I explained to him that fat takes up more room than muscle and that he should not be frustrated with the scale. His clothes will tell him everything about being thinner. After a few more weeks, the scale did start to show a lower number.

Many people, maybe even yourself, set expectations about the number on the scale, and when those expectations are not met, they quit, they give up. This might explain why people who make New Year's resolutions to exercise and lose weight stop after a few weeks. Many fail to keep up their workouts because they are not seeing immediate results. Or, their new exercise schedule and routine is not conducive to their family obligations, work responsibilities, and lifestyle.

It is not about the number on the scale,
It is about the inches of your waistline.

Exercise, however, is important for being fit and for overall health and wellness. Once you shed many of your extra pounds you will most likely want to be more physically active and begin an exercise program.

Thomas Edison said, "The doctor of the future will give no medicine but will interest his patients in the care of the human frame, in diet and in the cause and prevention of disease." Edison was wrong. The future is now, yet we consume more highly processed and manufactured foods that are scientifically engineered and full of chemicals. These foods are addictive and deadly. Furthermore, technology allows us to do fewer physical activities, i.e., getting off the couch to change the TV channel because we have remote controls, spending more time on computers and watching TV than playing outside, and the political climate which limits children from playing outdoors and having physical education classes.

More people are taking medications for preventable diseases and ailments. It's the new normal. I challenge you to be the exception. It's not about my being right or wrong. It's about what you will do. Will you be a part of the new normal or dare to be different?

I realize the information presented here might not be for everyone. However, you may know someone, perhaps a spouse, a friend, a colleague, an uncle, aunt, niece, or nephew who can benefit from the information. If you do, please share this information. It might just save a life like it saved mine.

"People are fed by the food industry, which pays no attention to health, and are treated by the health industry, which pays no attention to food."

– Wendell Berry

The Word **FATAL** has "Fat" in it.

Fatal means causing or capable of causing death; mortal, deadly, lethal.

Auto accidents, drug overdoses, and gun accidents combined do *not* account for a third of the deaths caused by food.

A recent study reveals that deaths due to excess body fat and obesity have now overtaken smoking-related deaths in people older than 45. Sitting and excessive eating are the new smoking habits.

Did you know that 90 percent of heart attacks are preventable through diet and physical activity, something as simple as walking every day.

The Chef and His Daughter

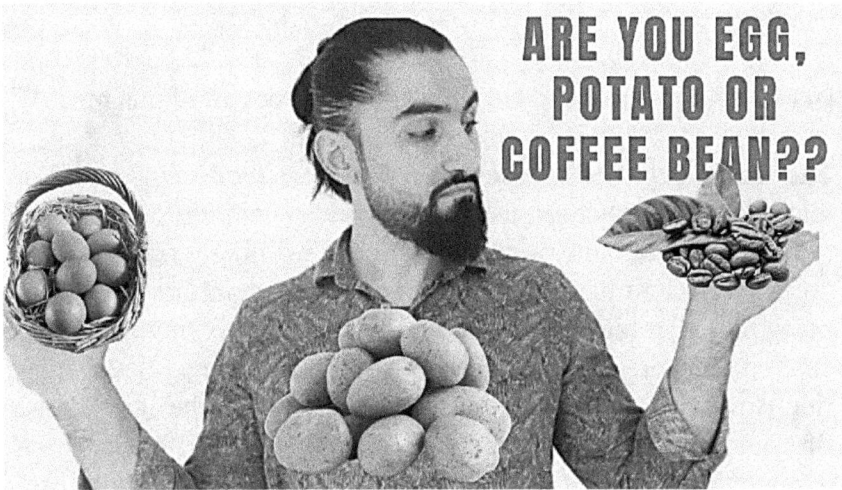

ARE YOU EGG, POTATO OR COFFEE BEAN??

There once was a girl who constantly complained to her father that her life was so hard and that she didn't know how she would get through all of her struggles. She was always tired. She believed that as soon as one problem was solved, another would arise. Does this sound familiar to you?

Being a chef, the girl's father took her into his kitchen. He boiled three pots of water that were equal in size. He placed potatoes in one pot, eggs in another, and ground coffee beans in the final pot. He let the pots boil, not saying anything to his daughter.

After twenty minutes he turned the burners off. He removed the potatoes from the pot and put them in a bowl. He did the same with the boiled eggs. Next, he used a ladle to scoop out the boiled coffee and poured it in a mug. He then asked his daughter, "What do you see?"

She responded, "Potatoes, eggs, and coffee."

Her father told her to take a closer look and touch the potatoes. After doing so, she noticed they were soft. Her father then told her to break open an egg. She did so and recognized the hard-boiled egg. Finally, he told her to take a sip of the coffee. It was rich and delicious.

Confused, the girl asked her father, "What does all of this mean?"

The father explained, "Each of these three food items had just undergone the exact same hardship–twenty minutes inside a pot of boiling water. However, each item had a different reaction. The potato went into the water as a strong, hard item, however after being boiled, it turned soft and weak. The egg was fragile when it entered the water, with a thin outer shell protecting a liquid interior. However, after it was left to boil, the inside of the egg became firm and strong. The ground coffee beans were different. Upon being exposed to boiling water, they changed the water to create something new altogether."

He then asked his daughter, "Which are you? When you face adversity, do you respond by becoming soft and weak? Do you build strength? Or do you change the situation?"

Your health journey will be full of ups and downs, wins and losses, and big shifts in momentum. Adversity will be a big part of your experience. While you would probably rather not encounter any difficulties, it doesn't always have to be a negative thing. You determine how you respond to the issues. Will you let it break you down? Will you stand up and meet the challenge or obstacle head-on? Or will you learn from it to improve your eating habits?

What is important to remember is when confronting adversity along your health quest, you have the freedom to choose how you respond. You can respond in a way that ultimately limits you, or you can choose to have it empower you.

*"Nature, in order to be commanded,
must be obeyed."*
– Francis Bacon

Don't Always Believe What is Being Advertised

The food, pharmaceutical, diet, and weight-loss industries pay millions of dollars to psychologists and marketing experts to manipulate you into buying their products. Their efforts could be referred to as "Zohnerism." Journalist James K. Glassman coined the term "Zohnerism" to describe *"the use of a true fact to lead a scientifically and mathematically ignorant public to a false conclusion."*

Zohnerism is the twisting of simple facts to confuse you!

In 1997, 14-year-old Nathan Zohner presented his science fair project to his classmates, seeking to ban a highly toxic chemical from everyday use. The chemical in question? Dihydrogen monoxide.

Throughout his presentation, Zohner provided his audience scientifically correct evidence as to why this chemical should be banned. After his presentation, 43 out of the 50 of his classmates voted to ban this clearly toxic chemical, dihydrogen monoxide.

The problem, however, is dihydrogen monoxide typically isn't considered toxic at all.

Dihydrogen monoxide is simply H2O (water).

Nathan Zohner's experiment was not an attempt to ban water. Rather, it was an experiment to get a representation of how gullible people can really be. What is important to understand is that all of the facts used by Nathan Zohner to make his argument were 100 percent factually correct; he just manipulated all of the information in his favor by omitting certain details.

This is what the food, pharmaceutical, diet, and weight-loss industries are doing to mislead you.

We see labels telling us it's *low fat,* yet that same food is high in sugar. While it's true that sugary foods are "fat free," what the label fails to tell you is sugar *causes fat to form* inside your body later. Then there are all these vegan-friendly foods that sound healthy but are filled with chemicals, dyes, and artificial preservatives. Potato chips and Oreo Cookies are vegan foods!

It is always good to question health statements touted as fact. Too often there are many perceived facts perpetuated by certain groups and companies about health, dieting, and weight-loss, which are untruthful, fabricated, or inaccurate. Believing some of these may be inhibiting you from achieving long-term, sustainable optimal health.

There is a lot of conflicting information about being healthy, especially when it comes to nutrition. Most likely, if you tell someone you're trying to eat healthier, they'll have tips, suggestions, and ideas for you to do. Be wary. There are too many companies peddling products that don't work or methods that will not promote good health. To achieve optimal health, you must make lifestyle changes.

Agnotology. Dr. Robert Lustig, M.D. introduced me to this word. Agnotology is the study of intentional and purposeful culturally induced ignorance usually to sell a product, influence an opinion, or gain support, through the publication of inaccurate or misleading scientific data. Hmmm, sounds similar to Zohnerism.

Culturally generated ignorance is propagated by the media, social media, government agencies, and corporations through manipulative and deceitful marketing tactics and transmissions. This is especially true when it comes to the food we consume. Many of my clients believe they are eating healthy until they learn to read the ingredients listed in the Nutritional Fact Panels/Labels. There is a reason the ingredients are listed at the bottom in very fine print…the food companies do not want you to know what you are consuming.

Chris Van Tulleken offers great insight into what consumers are eating in his book, *Ultra Processed PEOPLE The Science Behind Food That Isn't Food.* I highly recommend and endorse you read this book.

When it comes to living a healthy life, one size does not fit all. What could work for you might not work for someone else. What worked for me, might not work for you. Just because a dietary regimen worked for your neighbor doesn't mean you will have the same results. Each of us is unique and different. We have different eating preferences, different habits, and different body chemistry. Instead of attempting to pigeonhole yourself, think about eating healthy and living a healthy life based on your likes and dislikes. If you don't like Brussel Sprouts or Kale don't eat them just because they are healthy. The reason being is if you don't enjoy it, you won't continue to eat them.

Being busy is no excuse
for living an unhealthy lifestyle.

The Famous Gandhi Sugar Story

A woman walks with her son many miles to see Gandhi. She is worried her son is eating too much sugar. She asks Gandhi: "Please, sir, can you tell my son to stop eating sugar."

Gandhi says, "Bring him back in two weeks." Disappointed, she takes her son home.

Two weeks later she makes the long journey again. Gandhi says to the boy, "you must stop eating sugar. It's very bad for you."

The woman is confused and asks, "Why did you want me to wait two weeks to bring back my son."

Gandhi said, "Because before I could tell your son to stop eating sugar, I had to stop eating sugar first."

The boy has such respect for Gandhi that he stops and lives a healthy life.

The leadership idea: Changing yourself might help more than telling others they have to change.

And further still, Gandhi said that by changing yourself, you will change how you feel and what actions you take. And so have a real impact on the world around you.

"Anima Sana In Corpore Sano"
"Sound Mind in a Sound Body"

Living a Healthy Life Requires a System, Not Just a Goal

A goal is a clear and explicit idea of what you want the end result to be. Don't get me wrong. Goals are important. However, you need a plan of action to achieve your goal. W. Edward Deming said, "A goal without a method is nonsense." Make certain you have a method to achieve your health goal. Antoine de Saint-Exupery said, "A goal without a plan is just a wish." Individuals who have successful health regimens take the time to create a plan. Attempting to be healthy without a plan is like going from A to Z without stopping in between.

Have you set a health and wellness goal without having a proven, reliable plan or system to accomplish it?

The *9 Simple Golden Rules* for living a healthy life help you to create new eating routines which then become new behaviors and eventually new habits. And your new habits become a new way of life. You can never own your health and wellness success. You can only rent it. And the rent is due every day in the form of the food and beverage choices you choose to eat and drink.

People who are successful at eating healthy and living a healthy lifestyle are clear about their intentions. Those who fail are generally vague or uncertain.

For example, if you decide to reduce your soda or diet soda intake and drink more pure water, set a target to drink one-half of your daily soda intake while increasing your water intake. Achieving the smaller objectives does three things:

- Provides a systematic process
- Creates a sense of accomplishment
- Gives you small victories to celebrate

Achieving results, no matter how small, helps to keep you on course and encourages you to stay motivated to make healthy choices.

Start small and create a win for yourself. When you do this, you build confidence. With confidence you gain momentum. With momentum, you take more action to move closer to your goal. Nothing sustains motivation more than a sense of accomplishment.

Just because you reach a milestone and hit your number does not mean that you should stop attempting to keep improving yourself. Strive to improve every day.

"I don't care how old I live!
I just want to be living while I am living."

— Jack LaLanne, The "Godfather" of Fitness

The Thoroughbred Horse and His Owner

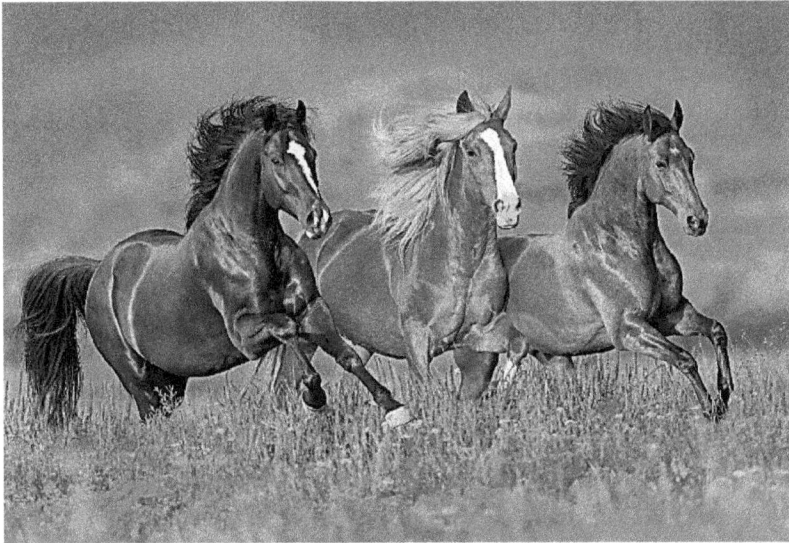

A few years ago, while in Las Vegas, I met the owner of a "prized" thoroughbred racehorse. During our conversation, he explained to me how he made certain his horse got the best nutritional supplements and ate the healthiest food to optimize the horse's performance. He boasted how he hired the best licensed and certified veterinarian to thoroughly examine the horse each week. He bragged about how the horse got the best dental care available.

The horse had his own personal trainer to exercise it every day. He made sure that the horse's environment was optimal for social interaction to keep the horse's spirits up. No expense was spared on maintaining the horse's health so the horse could perform at its best. Indeed, the man's knowledge about what the horse needed, and was provided, for optimal performance was remarkable.

However, what made the biggest impression on meeting this owner was how he cared for himself. You see, this gentleman was at least 75 pounds overweight. When the waiter served the owner's lunch, it was a huge hamburger loaded with cheese, bacon, lettuce and tomato, ketchup, mustard, and mayo. Of course, there was a side of golden French fries and an ice-cold Coke to wash down the food. It was apparent and obvious that this owner was more concerned about the health and care of his racehorse than himself.

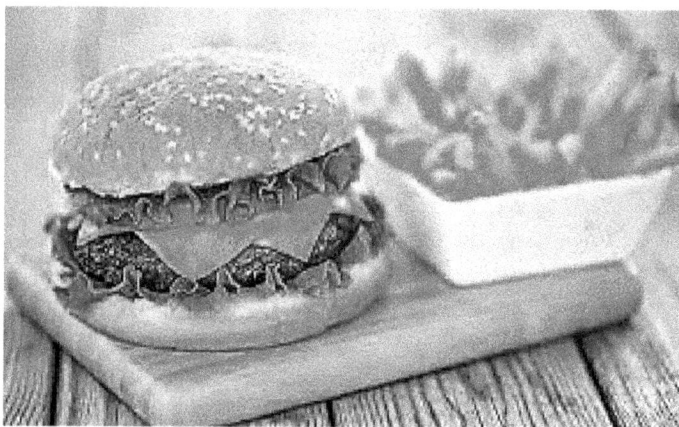

Pushing the conversation, I asked the owner how often he'd get a check-up from his doctor. The owner scoffed at the idea. His response, "I haven't been to a doctor in years. I'm as healthy as a horse." Uh-huh, I thought.

Now I'm certain you are thinking, I don't own a prized racehorse, so what's this got to do with me? Sadly, probably more than you realize. Do you own a pet, such as a dog or cat? If you do, most likely, you feed your dogs and pets more carefully than your own kids or yourself.

It's time to re-evaluate your health and fitness philosophy. There's a reason for the statement, "…is as healthy as a horse." Now is the time you should care for yourself like a prized racehorse so you can perform at your best.

TIP

Whenever possible, eat off a blue plate. The color blue is an appetite suppressant, whereas red and yellow are appetite stimulants.

That is probably why McDonald's, Wendy's, Burger King, KFC, Carl's Jr., and other fast-food places use red and yellow in their color schemes. The two largest pizza chains, Domino's Pizza, and Pizza Hut, both use red in their branding.

Routines, Behaviors, and Habits

It is the small, comfortable, daily steps toward change and improvement in your eating routine, behaviors, and habits that will give you success. You will not become healthy with abundant energy until you improve and change your eating routines. Routines become behaviors, and behaviors done consistently over a long time become new habits. A few habits may then become rituals. To be a ritual it must be sacred.

There's a major distinction between a habit and a ritual. Habits are done without thinking about them. They are automatic, such as brushing your teeth. Whereas a ritual is done with intention. Rituals generally reflect the values you've built into your life. Which means they are sacred to you. When you are creating something that's a reflection of your values and your purpose in your daily life, that's a ritual. For me, my morning ritual is to drink 20 ounces of pure water first thing. It's more than a habit because I do it intentionally.

Being healthy is not like getting a vaccination. You don't get one shot and forget about it. It doesn't work that way.

For a new behavior to happen consistently, you must find a way to remove all thinking, all discipline, and all willpower from the equation.

If you need to rely on any of that, you're screwed.

Have you experienced a lack of willpower or discipline?

Yeah, if you're being honest, you have, as seen from all your past New Year's resolutions, diets, and failed promises.

Improving your eating behaviors to become new habits will eliminate your need for self-control and willpower. Washing your
hands and face before you eat is a habit. You don't need self-control to wash your hands before you eat – you do it without thinking. A habit requires no decision-making because the decision has
already been made. With your improved eating habits, you don't
make decisions, you don't think, you just eat healthily because
that is how you eat.

The approach you will learn to change or create a habit is based
on the Keystone Habit discussed by Charles Duhigg in his book,
The Power of Habit, whereby changing one key habit can change
your entire life. A Keystone Habit is more important than others because it leads to the development of other habits. While
Keystone Habits don't necessarily create a direct cause-and-effect
relationship, they start a chain effect that produces other positive
outcomes.

Charles Duhigg told the story how Paul O'Neill changed one
Keystone Habit to transform the American Aluminum Company
of America, also known as ALCOA, a corporation that manufac-
tures everything from the foil that wraps Hershey's Kisses and the
metal in Coca Cola cans to the bolts that hold satellites together,
into an extremely profitable organization and a mainstay of safety.

According to Duhigg, shortly after Paul O'Neill became the new
CEO of ALCOA, he told Wall Street investors and stock analysts,
"I want to talk to you about worker safety. Every year, numerous ALCOA workers are injured so badly that they miss a day of
work. I intend to make ALCOA the safest company in America. I
intend to go for zero injuries."

The investors and analysts were confused. A new CEO normally talks about profit margins, new markets, and collaboration.
O'Neill said nothing about profits. He didn't mention any of the
usual talking points.

Eventually, someone asked about inventories in the aerospace division. Another asked about the company's capital ratio. O'Neill responded, "I'm not certain you heard me. If you want to understand how ALCOA is doing, you need to look at our workplace safety figures. Profits do not matter as much as safety."

When the presentation ended, the investors and analysts couldn't leave fast enough. One advisor immediately called twenty of his largest clients and told them, "There's a crazy hippie in charge who is going to kill the company." He advised them to sell ALCOA stock right away.

Within a year, however, ALCOA profits rose to record highs. By the time O'Neill left ALCOA in 2000 to become Treasury Secretary, annual net income for ALCOA was five times larger than before he arrived.

O'Neill transformed ALCOA into an extremely profitable organization by tackling one strategic area: safety—a Keystone Habit. That single change to improve safety rippled throughout the entire organization.

O'Neill said, "I knew I had to transform ALCOA. But you can't order people to change." This same concept applies to living a healthy life. We all know what to do – we just don't do it. No one can order or command you to change your eating habits and behaviors.

As to mandating people to conform with his directions, O'Neill said, "That's not how the brain works. I decided I was going to start by focusing on one thing. If I could start disrupting the habits around one thing, it would spread throughout the entire company."

This can work for you in your personal life and your journey to achieve optimal health. Simply pick one Keystone Habit or one key behavior to change. Focus on improving one thing. It could be one aspect of the food or beverages you eat or drink or one behavior you do while eating a meal. Just pick one to start, such as drinking water instead of soda or diet soda.

When you focus on changing and improving one key habit, it will have a ripple effect on your body, mind, and spirit, and positively affect almost every other aspect of your life.

"People don't die of old age.
They die of neglect."

– Jack LaLanne, The "Godfather" of Fitness

The Ripple Effect and Your Health

Based on a story told by Darren Hardy

One day a troubled team member knocked on the door to his boss's office and asked if he could talk with her for a moment. She invited him in and motioned for him to sit down.

The team member begins complaining about how the other team members don't like him, don't trust him, how they won't assign him any of the vital tasks, and how they don't invite him to the important meetings. The boss listens intently. The team member finishes his rant and asks the boss, "Will you speak to them about it?"

The boss asks the team member to join her on a walk. They walk to a pond in the middle of the office campus. The boss asks the team member to toss a stone into the center of the pond. The team member does as was asked.

Now she says, "As the ripples come closer to the shore, stick your hand in the water to stop the ripples."

The team member makes a valid attempt; however, he is unable to stop the ripples. The confused team member looks at his boss and exclaims, "I can't! It's impossible to stop the ripples."

The boss smiles and asks, "So, you are unable to stop the ripples?"

"Correct," said the team member.

"Well neither can I," said the boss. She continued, "I am unable to stop the ripples that you have created." She went on to explain,

"It's important for you to understand that every behavior, every action, every reaction, or comment you make creates a ripple. A ripple that will emanate throughout your entire pond. Throughout your entire team. All you can do is control what type of stone you throw to determine what ripple effect it will have. Is it a stone of encouragement? Is it a stone of support, contribution, or productivity? Or is it a stone of criticism or complaint? Is it a stone of doubt or dismissiveness or detraction?

What's beautiful about this is you will always get the effect of the stone you throw. And, even more incredible is the effect of the ripple as it spreads farther and wider than you intended or imagined. The stone of your comment or behavior doesn't affect the area where it enters the pond, it ripples throughout the rest of the pond, the rest of your team, maybe the rest of our client network."

What is the take-away lesson as it relates to your health?

It means that your food choices and lifestyle will have a ripple effect on your entire life.

Let me explain. It's important for you to understand that your lifestyle, every behavior, every action, every food, or beverage you choose to eat, or drink creates a ripple in your body. **A ripple that will emanate throughout your entire body and throughout your entire life.** All you can do is control what type of stone, i.e., the food and beverages you consume, and the lifestyle you live, to determine what ripple effect it will have. Is it a stone of health that fights disease? Is it a stone that supports your immune system, which improves your health, increases your energy, or enhances your mental clarity? Or is it a stone that weakens your immune system, causes you to have disease and illness, or makes your feel tired with little or no energy?

What's beautiful about this is you will always get the effect of the stone you throw. And, even more incredible is the effect of the ripple as it spreads farther and wider than you ever intended or imagined. The stone of your food choices, lifestyle, and behavior doesn't affect only your health, it ripples throughout your entire life. It affects your health, how you feel and look, your mood, your attitude, your confidence, which then affects how you treat and interact with members of your family, your work colleagues, or your clients. It affects your financial situation if you need to visit your doctors or not, whether you need to take prescription medication or not, or miss time from work.

Consider this. A person with excellent health has a thousand dreams. A person with poor health has just one – to be healthy. Choose wisely!

The next time you want to eat a doughnut, piece of cake or pie, a candy bar, ice cream, Dorito's, chips, muffins, cupcakes, cookies, a burrito, or other fa[s]t foods, ask yourself. "What would a healthy person do?" Would a healthy person eat those types of foods or drink soda, diet soda, or fruit juices? Would a healthy person walk or take a cab? Would a healthy person use the stairs or take an escalator or elevator?

"Your body is your most priceless possession. You've got to take care of it."

—Jack LaLanne, The Godfather of Fitness

Habits are Like Tree Roots

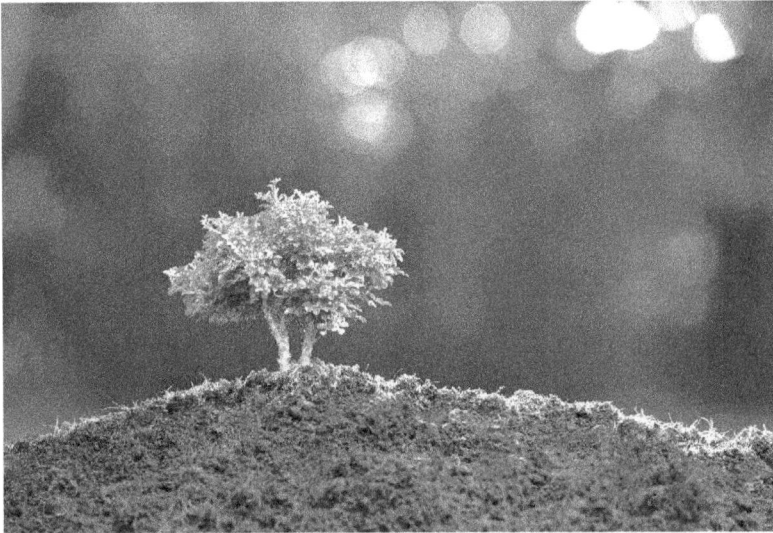

A wise woman was out walking in the forest with one of her young pupils. As they walked, they came across a young seedling that was just coming out of the ground. The wise woman asked the pupil to pull it out of the ground. The pupil did so with ease, and they walked on.

Shortly thereafter, they came upon a small tree. The wise woman asked her pupil to pull the small tree out of the ground. After struggling for about 45 minutes the pupil finally pulled the small tree from the ground. The two walked on.

As they walked, they came upon a mighty oak. The wise woman looked at her pupil, smiled, and instructed her pupil to remove the oak tree from out of the ground. The pupil stared at the mighty oak. He turned to the wise woman and said, "There is no way I can get this tree out of the ground. I was barely able to get the small tree out."

The woman responded, "So is the case with your habits, good or bad. The longer you let them grow, the deeper their root system becomes, and the taller they grow in your life. You might get to a point in your life where you don't think it's impossible to uproot them from your life. It's never too late to break a bad habit and create a good habit. It will, however, take more work and take longer to do. The lesson is not to allow bad habits to grow in your life."

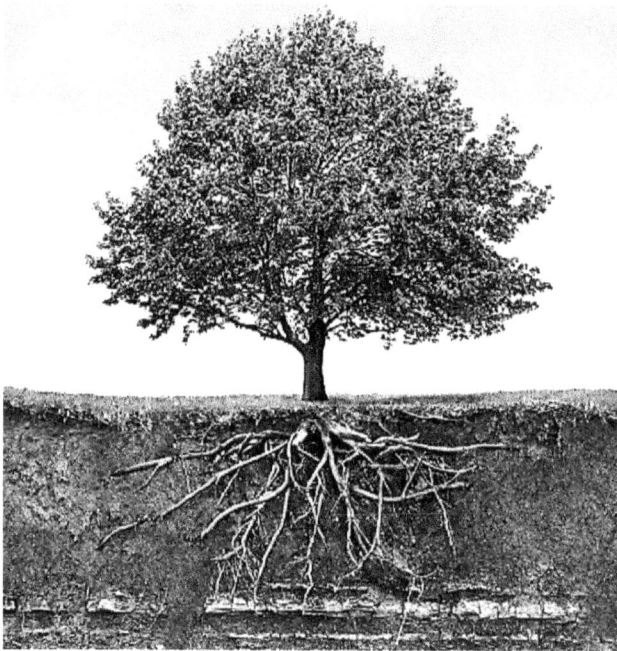

Requiem for the Employee

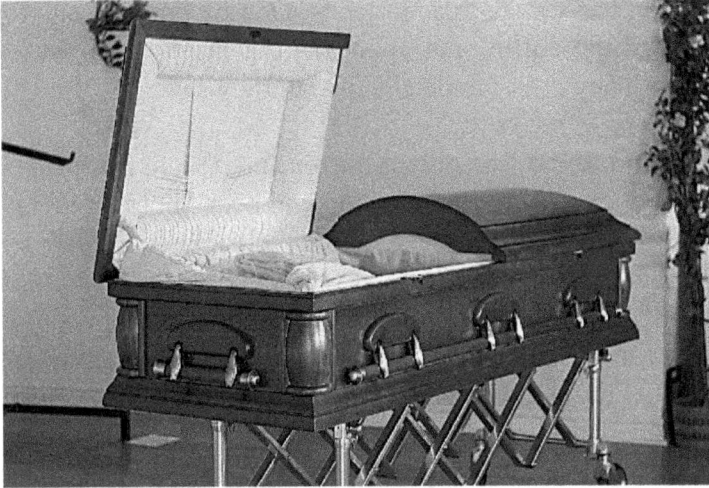

A CEO of a company, frustrated with the quality of work being done by his employees, started to discipline them for their mistakes or perceived lack of progress. However, nothing seemed to get the employees to improve their work ethics. The employees blamed the CEO for not being promoted to higher-paying positions within the company.

One day, as the employees came into work, they saw a sign on the door that read, "Yesterday, the person who has been holding you back from succeeding in this company passed away. Please gather for a funeral service in the assembly room."

The employees had assumed that the CEO had passed away. And, while they were saddened for the family of their CEO, they were also interested in the prospect of being able to now move up within the company and become more successful.

Upon entering the assembly room, many employees were stunned to see the CEO present. They wondered among themselves, "If it wasn't him who was holding us back from being successful, who was it? Who died?" The CEO asked each employee to pass by the open the coffin to pay their respects. One by one, the employees approached the coffin, and upon looking inside, each was quite surprised. They didn't understand what they saw.

In the coffin, there was only a mirror and a sign. So, when each employee looked in to find out who had been "holding them back from being successful" everyone saw themselves. Next to the mirror, there was a sign that read: The only person who is able to limit your growth is you. You are the only person who can influence your success. Your life changes when you break through your limiting beliefs and realize that you're in control of your life. The most influential relationship you can have is the relationship you have with yourself. Now you know who has been holding you back from living up to your true potential. Are you going to keep allowing that person to hold you back?

You are unable to blame anyone else except yourself if you are not as healthy and fit as you want to be. You have to take personal responsibility for your own health – the good and the bad. You are the only one who can be proactive in making improvements to your eating habits.

"If you don't like the road you're walking, start paving another one."

—Dolly Parton

EVERY DAY HEALTH CHOICES

THE 9 SIMPLE GOLDEN RULES FOR LIVING A HEALTHY LIFE

*"Health is a matter of choice.
Not a mystery of chance."*

– Aristotle

Based on thousands of hours of research, I have identified 9 Simple Golden Rules for every day health choices. They are:

1. Drink water.
2. Avoid fake foods.
3. Eat whole foods.
4. Eat slowly.
5. Eat small portions.
6. Sleep more.
7. Rest to digest.
8. Think positive.
9. Walk every day.

These are simple every day things that you CAN do.

Part of the reason you've been running into challenges of living a healthy lifestyle is because there's a difference between what you *CAN DO* and what you *WILL DO.* That's the distinction. It's not about what you can do, it's about what you will do.

Don't let the simplicity of the 9 Golden Rules fool you – They are game changers.

"When you ask another person to do something, it may help them if you tell them what to do, why they should do it, when they should do it, where they should do it, and how they may best do it."

– Napoleon Hill Foundation

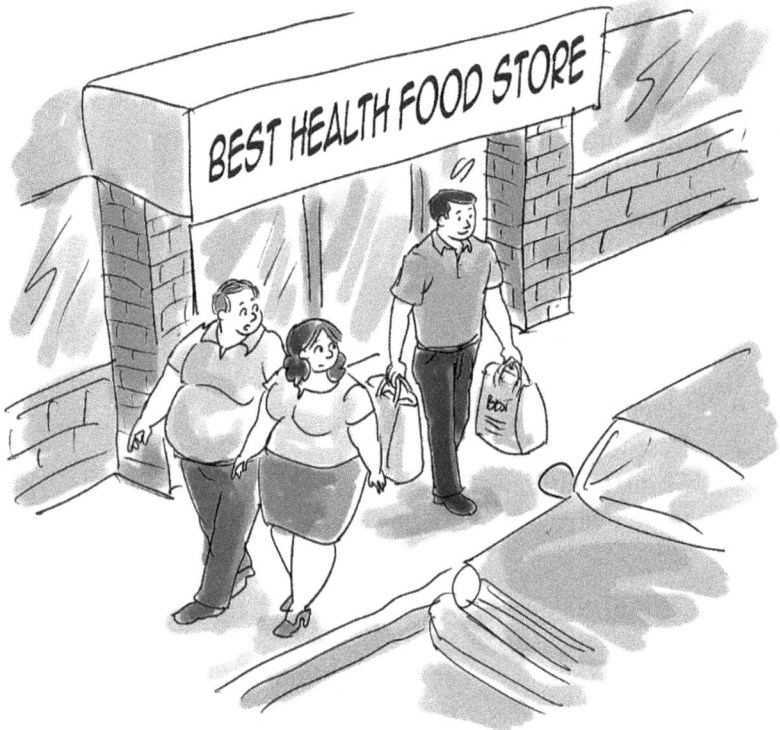

"POOR SCHMUCK, BOUGHT THAT HEALTH FOOD THING HOOK, LINE, AND SINKER."

Golden Rule Number One

DRINK WATER

The first golden rule is to drink an adequate amount (a minimum of 64 ounces) of pure water each day. However, it is advised that you drink one-half of your body weight in ounces of water. For example, if you weigh 200 pounds, drink 100 ounces of pure water, which is approximately twelve 8-ounce glasses.

Our bodies are made up of 60 to 70 percent water. Not soda, diet soda, fruit juice, or fruit flavored beverages – pure water. You wouldn't give your dog, cat, or other pets soda or diet soda to drink. Of course not.

Do you drink a minimum of 64 ounces of pure water each day?

Probably not.

How do I know this?

Because researchers found that more than 75 percent of the U.S. population suffers from chronic dehydration. In other words, seven out of ten people do not drink enough water. If you do nothing else, at least drink more pure water.

Americans are addicted to soda and diet soda. The average American drinks about 45 gallons of soda each year. Americans spend more money on soft drinks than any other beverage.

Did you know that much of the time when you think you're hungry, you're thirsty?

This could be one reason most of us eat too much. We should be drinking more pure water.

What do I mean by pure water?

Pure water, in my opinion, is distilled water, water processed by reverse osmosis, or spring water. It is not processed flavored waters. There is debate and dispute as to which is better between distilled water, reverse osmosis water, and spring water. Paul Bragg, ND, PhD., one of the original health crusaders, advocates that distilled water is best. However, his student, Jack LaLane believes spring water is better for you. And Dr. David Friedman, bestselling and award-winning author of *Food Sanity* feels that water filtered by a six-stage reverse osmosis system is best for you. I'll leave it up to your preference.

Drink water at room temperature because it is helpful in activating your digestive tract, improves circulation, aids in the digestive process, helps relieve constipation, flushes out toxins from your body, and much more. Also, drinking warm water first thing in the morning might help to jump-start your metabolism.

Cold water, on the other hand, could be detrimental because it can prevent your body from absorbing vitamins, minerals, and other nutrients. Your body's natural temperature is between 98.6- and 100.8-degrees Fahrenheit. When you drink a cold beverage, your body needs to exert a lot of energy to regulate your core temperature. This diverts energy away from the energy needed to digest your food and absorb nutrients. However, some experts believe you should drink cold water after exercising or other strenuous physical activities because it helps lower your body's core temperature quicker.

Cold water has been shown to increase your risk for headaches. According to a research study by Cephalalgia published in 2001 by the International Headache Society, drinking cold water was twice as likely to induce a headache in women who experienced migraines. Have you ever had "brain freeze" when you ate or drank something cold too quickly? Ouch!

Cold water (or any other cold beverage) may contain ice made from contaminated water. Recent studies found that the ice made in your freezer, store bought, or in beverages from restaurants, is full of bacteria, some of which is unhealthy.

If you think buying bottled water is safe, think again. Americans spend almost $17 billion each year on bottled water believing it's safe. However, the federal government does more testing and quality control on tap water than on bottled water.

Many brands of bottled water will mislead you and fool you into thinking their water is from underground springs or glaciers. It's B.S.! They are from municipal tap water. This includes two of the most popular brands, Aquafina, manufactured by PepsiCo, and Dasani, produced by Coca-Cola.

Who would have imagined that plain (not to be confused with pure) water with zero calories, zero carbs, zero fat, and zero sugar could be causing you to gain weight? Unfortunately, it is true.

So, what can you do to protect yourself from drinking contaminated water?

One suggestion is to invest in a water filtering system (not to be confused with a water filter) that removes these chemicals and heavy metals. However, it should not be just any water filtering system. It needs to be a six-phase reverse osmosis system with re-mineralization. There are several reverse osmosis systems with seven phases and ultraviolet (UV) light bulbs on the market. These are not recommended because UV light can heat the water to extremely hot temperatures. The high temperatures can weaken or loosen the fittings. Also, make certain the system has an NSF certification for removal of substance on the label.

An iSpring RCC7AK, NSF Certified 75 GPD, Alkaline 6-Stage Reverse Osmosis System, pH+ Remineralization RO Water Filter System Under Sink, Superb Taste Drinking Water Filter sells for about $220.

Once you have your reverse osmosis system operating, you can use a stainless-steel bottle, a durable BPA-free bottle, or a glass bottle to bring your water with you when you're not at home.

AVOID "FLAVORED" WATERS

The ingredients in Nestlé Splash Flavored Water, Lemon are: Purified Water, *Citric Acid*, Sodium Polyphosphate, Natural Flavors, Potassium Sorbate (Preserve Freshness), *Potassium Benzoate* (Preserve Freshness), Sucralose, Acesulfame Potassium, Calcium Disodium EDTA, and Magnesium Sulfate.

So, you might be thinking, what is the big deal?

When *potassium or sodium benzoate* is mixed with *citric acid*, it forms benzene. Benzene is a carcinogen associated with leukemia and other blood cancers.

Nestlé "purifies" their water and then adds all these unhealthy, disease-causing chemicals. Why? Because Nestlé has multi-billion-dollar partnerships with big chemical corporations. They make money from YOU, the consumer, and chemical corporation "side deals."

SUGGESTIONS ON HOW TO DRINK MORE WATER

- Upon rising, drink one to two eight-ounce glasses of water. (8 to 16 ounces)

- Drink one to two eight-ounce glasses of water mid-morning. (8 to 16 ounces)
- Drink one to two eight-ounce glasses of water before lunch. (8 to 16 ounces)
- Drink one to two eight-ounce glasses of water mid-afternoon. (8 to 16 ounces)
- Drink one to two eight-ounce glasses of water before dinner. (8 to 16 ounces)

This will help you to drink between 40 and 160 ounces of water each day.

Keep track of the water you drink either in a daily food journal or on a piece of paper, or cell phone. You might be drinking less water than you realize.

Golden Rule Number Two

AVOID FAKE FOODS

Golden rule number two is to avoid consuming highly processed and manufactured foods, also known as fake foods.

For decades food companies have scientifically engineered the packaged fake food you purchase in the grocery store to be addictive. They refer to these enhanced fake foods as the "Bliss Point."

The Bliss Point is a term coined by Howard Moskowitz for how food manufacturers add artificial ingredients and other chemicals to increase the optimization of the food's tastiness, automatically increasing your cravings for it. Simply stated, foods are developed to be so tasty it's hard to resist them. In other words, they are addicting. Food manufacturers are turning you into food junkies with the junk they are pushing on you just like a dealer pushes illegal drugs such as meth, opioids, and heroin to junkies. Did you know Oreo cookies are more addictive than cocaine? Imagine that. A cookie is more addictive than an illegal drug.

Consider this. In 1975 the average supermarket carried about 9,000 food products (SKUs = Stock Keeping Unit). Today, the average grocery store carries about 35,000 products with some carrying as many as 60,000 products. I don't know about you, I've not heard of many new fruits, vegetables, berries, or nuts being discovered during this time period. The reason there are so many more food products is from the rapid increase of highly processed foods with grains and manufactured foods being chemically engineered in labs.

How does this affect you?

Nutritionists say this creates an expectation that everything we eat should either taste sweet or salty. This is one explanation why kids rebel against eating fresh produce. To them it tastes sour or bitter. Unfortunately, because of these Bliss Point food products, the human body has evolved to crave foods that deliver just the right amount of saltiness, richness, and sweetness. That's because your brain responds with a reward in the form of endorphins. It remembers what you did to get that reward, and makes you want to do it again.

This is why you want to keep eating your fake foods even though you are full. It's an effect run by dopamine and neurotransmitters. Your mind will never be satisfied. You can never get enough—just like a junkie on heroin. Perhaps that's why it's referred to as junk food... because it makes you a food junkie.

When Lay's boasts "Bet you can't eat just one" about their potato chips, it's not a dare. It's a fact!

More Fake Foods: Meatless Meat—
Beefless Beef, Chicken-Less Chicken, Fishless Fish

The problem today is the biggest trend in the food industry has nothing to do with organic beef or free-range chicken. In fact, the juiciest burgers you might eat are made of pea protein and other chemicals.

Popular examples of plant-based beef include the Impossible Burger, the Beyond Burger, and the myriad of options now commonly found in the freezer section of the grocery store. Plant-based burgers are now sold in fast-food places such as McDonald's, Burger King, White Castle, Carl's Jr., and other fast-food places. Even respectable and expensive restaurants are serving the Impossible Burger with their own creative toppings.

Plant-based alternative meats also apply to chicken and sausages being manufactured to look and taste as close to chicken without harming a chicken (KFC's vegan fried chicken) or pig. While plant-based meats—beef, chicken, pork, and fish—are often heralded for tasting and looking like the real thing, many experts are still unsure if they are healthy. In my opinion, they are not because of the chemicals used to create these fake foods. Mother Nature did not create plants to look and taste like meat.

Chiffon was one of the first soft, tub-style margarine products sold as a butter substitute. In the 1970s, Chiffon ran television ads featuring Hollywood actress Dena Dietrich as Mother Nature, who mistook the Chiffon substitute for real butter. Her character's slogan, "It's not nice to fool Mother Nature," became a pop culture catchphrase. Perhaps today's consumer should heed these words as a warning.

Meatless meats and similar food substitutes aren't as good for you as you may think. You have to look at the ingredients and nutrition facts to find out exactly what you're eating. It is important to remember that these are still highly processed products. They are not whole foods – they are just part of a food.

Fake plant-based burgers include coconut and other oils, and each includes a host of ingredients such as methylcellulose, soy leghemoglobin, zinc gluconate, modified food starch, cultured dextrose, and soy protein isolate. This means the imitation (fake) meat is not a whole food created by nature. It is a manufactured food. Do not confuse real food created by nature with fake foods created in a lab by someone in a white lab coat. There is a difference.

It is ironic how many people are concerned about air pollution and water pollution yet have no qualms about polluting their own bodies with highly processed and chemically augmented manufactured fake foods which are produced by creating lots of air, water, and soil pollution.

"You can't fix your health until you fix your diet."

– Unknown

Golden Rule Number Three

EAT WHOLE FOODS

Golden rule number three is to eat whole, holistic foods, mostly plants, and organic if possible.

In today's fast-paced, high-demand world, our culture has focused on convenience, and that includes how we eat. When we are hungry, it's much easier to go to the drive-thru, open a can, unwrap a package or pop a lid than it is to prepare a fresh meal. However, the trade-off for convenience is that it has a dramatic impact on your health. The rise of obesity is a direct link to your health and what you eat has taken center stage.

What are holistic foods? Holistic food is as close to its natural state as possible for optimum health and well-being. Holistic foods include unrefined, unprocessed, organic, and whole foods that are locally grown. Holistic or whole foods are foods that have been grown and nourished from the earth rather than manufactured and sold in a box or foil package.

The contrast between these two kinds of foods lies in the difference in nutrient content. Fruits, vegetables, legumes, beans, nuts, seeds, and whole grains are a rich source of the vitamins and minerals that our bodies require.

Although processed foods may be enriched or enhanced with vitamins and minerals, they are rarely in the forms most bioavailable to our bodies. When you eat food that is vibrant and alive, you invite that vitality into your own body.

By choosing to eat more whole or holistic foods, you may experience health benefits, such as:

- Weight loss
- Increased energy levels
- Improved mood
- Better sleep
- Improved skin tone and texture
- Strengthened immune system
- Balanced blood sugar levels
- Reduced cholesterol and blood pressure levels
- Improved digestion and relief from constipation
- Additionally, you may lower your risk for chronic illnesses that can be prevented or improved through diet, such as:
- Type 2 diabetes
- Arthritis
- Heart disease
- High blood pressure
- Cancer
- Colitis
- Gout

Eating whole, raw food is the simplest way to provide your body with proper nourishment. For a healthy snack, eat an apple, banana, carrot, celery, grapes, melon, avocado, or your favorite fruit or vegetable the way nature intended—raw and unprocessed. Another thing you can do is eliminate white flour or white rice because the white varieties are stripped of most of their nutrition and fiber. Other suggestions for eating whole foods and accomplish an eating behavior improvement and change:

- Eat cherries and unsalted/raw nuts as a snack. *Unless, of course, you are allergic to nuts.* Then you might consider berries (fresh or frozen) such as strawberries, blueberries, raspberries, or blackberries.

- Eat green leafy vegetables for salad and avoid high-fat/high-caloric salad dressings.
- Eat an orange instead of drinking a glass of orange juice.
- Avoid fried foods.

Unfortunately, most of us have a SAD food intake. SAD, which stands for Standard American Diet, is the primary cause of chronic disease and illness. But no matter how much evidence exists on the health benefits of eating a mostly plant-based diet, the fact remains that most Americans will never give up their processed foods and SAD, fast food, lifestyle. Will you?

If you're serious about changing the foods you eat, avoid eating store-bought bread or bread used to make sandwiches at fast-food places. For an alternative, eat Ezekiel bread. Ezekiel bread is made using an assortment of sprouted grains. The sprouted grains increase the nutritional value of the bread. And, unlike other store-bought breads that can last on a shelf for months, Ezekiel bread must be refrigerated or frozen; otherwise, it spoils quickly.

It is more than just calories in and calories out when you're attempting to reduce weight in a healthy manner that's sustainable. It's about the quality of the calories you consume because not all calories are equal in nutritional benefits. Achieving and maintaining a healthy weight is about choices. We all have choices. Why wait until you're in a health crisis if it can be avoided?

"If this country is to survive, the best-fed-nation myth had better be recognized for what it is: propaganda designed to produce wealth but not health."

—Adelle Davis

Golden Rule Number Four

EAT SLOWLY

Golden rule number four is to eat slowly.

There is value to eating slowly. It's one of the simplest yet most powerful things you can do to improve your overall health. We're all rushed, distracted, and too busy. Most people in the United States eat fast. Really fast. Rarely do people take the time to savor their food – or sometimes even to chew it properly.

Eating slowly allows your body time to recognize that you're full. It takes about 20 minutes from the time you start to ingest your meal for the brain to signal you that you're satisfied. Most meals don't even last that long. As you learned from Golden Rule 2, food is scientifically engineered so that our brain never gets the signal to stop eating.

Eating slowly helps you feel satisfied before overeating. Imagine the extra calories, sugars, carbs, and fats you could eliminate simply by eating slower. Marc David, author of *The Slow Down Diet*, suggests if you eat breakfast in five minutes, increase the time to 10. If you normally take 10 minutes, increase it to 15 or 20. Give yourself a minimum of 30 minutes (a half hour) for lunch and dinner.

Eating quickly leads to poor digestion, increased weight gain, and lower gratification. Eating slow advances improved digestion, better hydration, easier weight-loss or maintenance, and greater enjoyment of our meals. Slow down your eating to enjoy your food. This will also promote your overall health and well-being.

Shoveling down your food means that you can sneak in a lot of extra calories before your stomach realizes what is going on.

Here are a few suggestions to help you slow down your eating behavior:

- Put the fork or spoon down between each bite.
- Avoid eating while driving.
- Avoid eating while working or at your desk.
- Avoid eating while watching television.
- Focus on eating and enjoying your food.
- Avoid distractions while eating. This can cause "mindless" eating.

MINDLESS EATING

Mindless eating refers to an eating behavior where calories are consumed while the individual is unaware of the quantity being eaten or that he/she is eating in the first place.

Mindless eating can occur any time that your brain is distracted, and you are not aware of what or how much food you are consuming.

Mindless eating usually happens while another activity is going on simultaneously.

Mindless eating occurs when you're not aware that you just consumed an entire pint of ice cream or devoured a full bag of potato chips or other snacks because you weren't paying attention to the food you were stuffing into your mouth while focusing on other things.

Here are a few examples:

- Watching TV and eating chips out of a bag and before you know it half the bag is gone. Watching television detrimentally affects your eating habits, which can cause obesity. Studies show a direct correlation between watching television and weight gain.

- Sitting at work in front of the computer while the bowl of candy nearby slowly disappears, unintentionally.
- Eating popcorn out of the bucket at the movies and munching away while you're engrossed by the film.

Where Do You Eat Your Meals?

- At the kitchen table?
- In front of your computer?
- While watching TV?
- In your car driving?
- At your desk in your office or at work?
- A restaurant?

Where you eat might increase the quantity you consume. Consider consciously changing the location of your meals.

There are several other factors that contribute to mindless eating. Some of these are:

- **Boredom**. Eating when you're not hungry because you are bored and eating food or snacks is going to give you something to do.
- **Distracted eating**. You are eating when your mind is sidetracked by television, working, driving, watching a movie, or other diversions.
- **Awareness**. Overeating because you are unaware just how much food you are consuming because you are eating directly out of the bag or box, or not measuring portion sizes. As an example, grabbing a few handfuls of nuts out of the can or jar. Each handful could have as many as 100 calories each.

- **Emotions.** Some individuals turn to food for comfort when they are sad, anxious, upset, hurt, or angry.
- **Commercials and advertisements.** An outside source, such as food advertisements or television commercials.

Have you noticed that commercials displayed on the TV screen during prime time and late at night are prominently for food and restaurants? They're designed and created to entice you to eat more. Further, eating late at night is the worst time to chow down. To add insult to injury, the advertisements usually depict thin people. If you have a poor self-image, you might consume more food to comfort yourself.

WHAT YOU CAN DO TO COMBAT A TELEVISION EATING HABIT

- Do a few push-ups between commercials. The average commercial break is two to five minutes. Instead of getting up to grab a snack, do some push-ups. Even if you start with five. You can build up to doing 25 to 50 push-ups during a commercial break.
- Do some leg lifts. Again, start slowly and build up. Before you know it, you'll be doing 25 to 50 leg lifts during each commercial break along with your push-ups.
- Not fond of leg lifts? Do squats. Or grab light-weight dumbbells. There are many things you can do during a commercial break to get some physical activity. Imagine, you won't need to go to the gym to do a workout. You'll save time and money.

The average one-hour television show has between seven and 10 commercial breaks. If you can build up to doing just 25 push-ups during just four commercial interruptions, you'll have done 100 push-ups during the show. Do it gradually if you haven't done much or any exercise in a while.

Track how many hours you spend watching television. It may surprise you how much time you're wasting in front of the screen. With Netflix and other subscription channels, there are no commercials. And during the COVID-19 pandemic, these subscription networks gained millions of new viewers.

It's important to be aware of just how many hours you are sitting in front of the boob tube without moving!

WHAT ELSE CAN YOU DO TO CURTAIL MINDLESS EATING?

Pre-portion your servings. For example, instead of grabbing a handful of nuts, count out 10. Eat them slowly, one at a time, instead of putting the entire handful into your mouth. Avoid eating while watching television. If you do eat or snack while watching TV, don't eat out of the bag. Instead, portion out an individual serving into a small bowl.

Avoid eating your meals such as dinner or lunch while working at your desk or in front of your computer. Take at least 30 minutes to eat lunch and 30 minutes to eat dinner. Focus on the food you are consuming.

Avoid eating while driving. If you choose to go through the drive-thru at a fast-food place, park and eat your meal before driving to your destination.

Track your eating behavior for a few weeks. Then look for patterns. If it appears there's a relationship between eating and feelings, think of ways to meet emotional needs without turning to food.

Ask people in your support community for suggestions. Connect with an accountability buddy you can talk to, so you avoid comfort eating. Maybe take a walk, or you can do some yoga or other quick exercises.

MINDFUL EATING

So, the opposite of "mindless" eating is "mindful" eating. Mindful eating is a method that allows you to gain control over your eating habits.

To be a mindful eater means that you are fully aware of the food you are eating, how much you are consuming, and the ability to really enjoy and savor the flavor of the food.

Tips To Become A Mindful Eater:

- Eat slower. When you slow down, appreciate a meal, notice the food's tastes and textures, you'll enjoy each bite. This one small adjustment to your current eating routine can help you lose weight.
- Think about why you are eating. Is it because you are hungry or is it because you are bored? Maybe you are upset, anxious, or excited?
- If at all possible, eat your meals at a kitchen or dining room table.
- Pay attention to what you are eating, and how much you are eating.
- As best you can, enroll your family, co-workers, and boss in creating more time and relaxation with meals. Find a "slow down" buddy to share meals and encourage each other to slow down while eating.
- Eat only in a sitting position.
- Choose not to answer your cell phone, home phone, or texts while eating.

Golden Rule Number Five

EAT SMALL PORTIONS

Golden rule number five is to eat small portions.

Did you know your food portions have been supersized without you knowing it?

It's true. The average dinner plate in the 1900s was nine inches in diameter. Over the years, plate sizes have been made larger. In 2000, the diameter of the average-size dinner plate was 11 inches. Today, the diameter of the average-size dinner plate is 12 inches. Yet in Europe, the diameter of the average-size dinner plate is still nine inches. Perhaps this is one of the reasons that the United States has a weight problem.

Restaurants are notorious for giving portions that are two or three times more than what we should be eating. In restaurants, the diameter of the average serving plate is 13 to 15 inches. This means you are consuming almost 75 percent more food than is necessary.

So, what can you do when the server brings you your food that is too much to eat at one sitting? Simply cut it in half and ask for a to-go box. Put one-half in the to-go box. This will help you from overeating. Plus, you'll save money. It's like getting two meals for the price of one. Or you can split a meal with your spouse, friend, or significant other.

So, what can you do to reduce your food portions at home? Use a salad plate instead of a dinner plate. If you put the exact amount of food on a salad plate as on a dinner plate, the food on the dinner plate will look like you're getting less, and the food on the salad plate will look like you're getting more. It's an optical illusion. It's known as the Delboeuf Illusion.

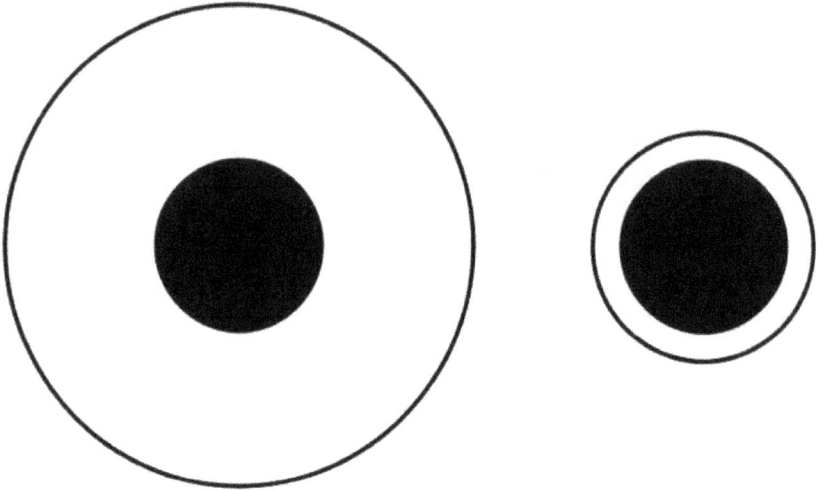

Franz Joseph Delboeuf, a Belgian mathematician and philosopher, first documented this phenomenon in 1865. Delboeuf started with two dots of equal size. He surrounded one dot with a large circle and the other dot with a small one. He noticed the second dot looked bigger.

Research suggests that choices, like how much to eat during a meal, are often made subconsciously. The problem arises because our brains are hardwired to mislead us in lots of little ways, which can have a big impact on our diets.

Researchers also measured serving behavior in the real-world atmosphere of a buffet line. They found the same results. People underserved on small dishes, while the reverse was true and over-estimated for large dishes. People using the smallest dishes under-shot the target serving by as much as 12 percent. However, people using the largest dishes took up to 13 percent more food than they intended.

MAGIC WORDS TO USE WHEN DINING OUT

You can control your portions while dining out. These are the magic words you can use when eating at a restaurant. Inform the server, "I am on a restricted diet. I'd like to order…a plain grilled chicken breast with a side of avocado," or "a grilled salmon with a side of steamed broccoli," or "a grilled steak (6 ounces or smaller) with a side of plain green beans/mixed green salad (with dressing on the side)," etc. Every time I've done this, the server has been more than willing to accommodate my request.

The beauty of this is that the server does not need to know why you are on a restricted diet. They do not know if you are attempting to lose weight, have food allergies, or any other reason. Not one server has ever asked me the reason.

It has been scientifically proven that the size of your dinnerware affects your behavior for how much food you consume. Consider this: if you increase your caloric intake by just 50 calories per day because you're eating more than you should, you will gain an additional five pounds within one year.

This is how the weight creeps up on us. It's gradual over a long period of time. Imagine reversing that trend and eating less simply by using a smaller plate. You'd most likely reduce your caloric intake by 50 calories per day. Which means, over time, you'd get rid of extra weight.

As you will recall, if you shed just two pounds per month on average for 12 consecutive months, you'd weigh 24 pounds less within one year. The opposite holds true. This is why the size of your serving plate matters.

PORTIONS (HOW MUCH SHOULD I EAT?)

To help you determine the appropriate portion size for you and your body as it relates to protein, complex carbohydrates, and healthy fats—without using measuring cups, food scales, or other calorie-counting devices—use this quick reference guide:

- The palm of your hand determines the size of how much protein you should eat.
- Your fist determines the portion size of how much vegetables you should eat (although you can eat as many raw or steamed vegetables as you desire).
- Your cupped hand defines the portion size of complex carbohydrates you should consume, and
- Your thumb defines how much healthy fat you can consume.

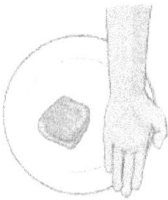

A portion of protein = 1 palm   A portion of vegetables = 1 fist   A portion of carbs = 1 cupped hand   A portion of fats = 1 thumb

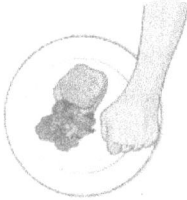

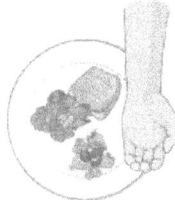

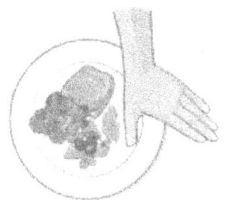

Counting Calories – No Need to Do It

For most people, counting calories does not work for delivering sustainable, healthy weight-loss. Based on the experience of thousands of folks, there are several problems with counting calories. These include but are not limited to:

The number of calories is meaningless to most people. If calories meant anything, people would avoid eating many of the meals listed on the menu at restaurants. When was the last time you paid attention to the calories shown on a menu?

The calories do not distinguish between healthy foods and unhealthy foods. As an example, a regular size Hershey's chocolate bar has about 125 calories. An apple has about 100 calories. The apple provides more fiber and nutritional value than the Hershey's bar. Plus, your body will burn about 25 calories to digest the apple, where it takes zero calories to digest the Hershey's bar.

The number of calories is often wrong. The number of calories in a food item is an estimate. That estimate can be off by as much as 20 percent.

The number of calories does not factor in the impact of other eating behaviors such as where a person is eating, when a person is eating, or how fast a person is eating.

Counting calories can create additional emotional, psychological, and mental issues for people. The point about counting calories is that it will *not* help you improve your eating behaviors and develop a healthier lifestyle. It might even thwart your relationship with food.

glut·ton·y

/ˈɡlət(ə)nē/

noun

- habitual greed or excess in eating.

Gluttony means over-indulgence and over-consumption of food or drink.

Golden Rule Number Six

SLEEP MORE

Golden rule number six is to sleep more.

Researchers have found that getting adequate sleep each night is a basic principle for maintaining good health and lowering your risk of gaining weight.

Why?

Because not getting the proper amount of sleep elevates your cortisol levels. Cortisol causes your body to go into fat storage mode. Elevated cortisol levels cause junk food cravings. In addition, not having enough sleep makes you tired, which increases your cravings for sugary and simple carbohydrate foods. You'll know if you're tired all the time because you'll also be hungry all the time.

Getting adequate sleep is crucial for reducing weight. Getting enough sleep is required for turning off your body's fat-retention programs, reducing stress, lowering cortisol levels, and maintaining proper hormonal balance.

You need to get adequate sleep to successfully reduce weight. According to an article titled, *Sleep and Weight Loss*, written by Dr. Muhammad Usman, M.D. for weightlossresources.co.uk, the average person who is sleep deprived will consume an extra 385 calories per day. It takes an average of reducing 500 calories per day for an entire week to lose one pound. Think about that. You're going in the wrong direction without adequate sleep.

It is better, for weight-loss purposes and overall health, to take a nap in the afternoon instead of exercising or working out. That is, you will lose more weight by taking a nap in mid-afternoon than you will if you work out. I know it sounds contradictory to what we've been taught; however, if you are sleep deprived, it's better to take a nap. Nothing is more important than getting the proper amount of sleep when you're tired and when you're attempting to reduce weight.

BEHAVIOR CHANGES FOR SLEEPING BETTER AT NIGHT:

- Turn your computer screens off an hour before bedtime.
- Turn your television off an hour before bedtime.
- Turn your Wi-Fi on your phone off at bedtime.
- Put your phone in airplane mode.
- Make the room as dark as possible.
- Keep the room cool. Studies show that when a room is cool you sleep better.

Do you watch television in your bedroom? This can disrupt sleep and cause other health issues. Research shows that the nighttime glow streaming from the television throws off biorhythms, messes with hunger signals, and has a direct correlation to weight gain. In addition, the TV emits dangerous substances from many of its materials when it is warm. A simple solution is to remove the problem from the bedroom or make certain it has been off an hour before you go to sleep.

Here's the honest truth about people who judge you: They're trying to discourage you so that you feel as bad as they do. That's their problem. Don't make it yours by letting what they say impact what you do."

—Mel Robbins

Golden Rule Number Seven

REST TO DIGEST

Golden rule number seven is to give your body time each day to digest and process the food you consume. You may want to do intermittent fasting.

Whenever fasting is mentioned, there is always the same eye-rolling response. Starvation. Can you relate to this?

Did you roll your eyes, too?

Have you seen the ads and online messages about intermittent fasting?

With all the hype about it, you may feel it's just another modern diet fad. The truth is fasting is thousands of years old.

Fasting is not starvation. Starvation is the involuntary absence of food. It is neither deliberate, nor controlled. Starving people have no idea when and where their next meal will come from.

Fasting is the voluntary withholding of food for spiritual, health, or other reasons. The two terms, "starvation" and "fasting" should never be confused with each other. In a sense, fasting is part of everyday life. The term "break-fast" is the meal that breaks the fast, which, for many people, is done daily by eating breakfast cereal or a breakfast sandwich. My question is, "Who said you must eat breakfast cereal as the first meal of the day?"

The reality is that it's the cereal companies promoting the myth that you must eat cereal for breakfast. The truth is that you can eat anything you want for breakfast.

Fasting means giving your body a rest period to digest the food you consume.

Fasting is one of the oldest and most well-known healing rituals in the world. Hippocrates, who is widely considered the father of modern medicine, prescribed the practice of fasting as treatments. Hippocrates wrote, "To eat when you are sick is to feed your illness."

Fasting isn't abnormal. It's a natural healing process. Fasting is widespread. Fasting remains part of virtually every major religion in the world. Jesus Christ, Buddha, and the prophet Muhammed all shared a common belief in the power of fasting for cleansing or purification.

In other words, healing.

It's only until recently in human history that people have not gone for extended periods of time without food. Throughout our evolutionary history, there would be periods lasting days, weeks, or months during which food resources were scarce.

Today, in our modern society, we are blessed, or cursed depending on the source, with an abundance of food. Unfortunately, much of our food today is manufactured, highly or ultra processed. We overconsume products full of sugar, dairy, and grains that are high in calories and unhealthy fats. Yet with all this overconsumption, our bodies do not get enough nutrients. It's these ultra processed and manufactured food products that generate unhealthy behaviors, such as poor diet, and promote the chronic disease epidemic. In essence, individuals are suffering from chronic illnesses because of product environment wherein companies are putting their profits over your health.

Dr. Peter Osborne, the clinical director at Origins Healthcare in Sugarland, Texas, and author of the best-selling book *No Grain, No Pain*, provides a great analogy. Dr. Osborne says to imagine that you go home from work every day and prepare your meals, eat, but never do your dishes. The dishes keep piling up in the sink. Eventually, they start spilling out of the sink and onto the countertop. Before you know it, you have bugs eating the debris of the food left on the dishes. And you have a huge mess in your house because you didn't do the dishes.

Dr. Osborne says that's what happens in your stomach. When you put too much in and don't have normal "housekeeping," the stomach becomes overwhelmed, and your gastrointestinal system becomes a breeding ground for bacteria. And when you eat all the time and don't give your stomach a rest, it becomes exhausted. Your gut needs a vacation!

This is where fasting comes in. You're giving your body a chance to clean the dishes, so to speak. It gives your body a chance to rest and repair itself.

My friend and naturopathic doctor Rachel Smartt had this analogy to explain the importance of fasting. Dr. Smartt describes fasting as your body being a power lawn mower and the food you consume being wet grass. As you mow wet grass, it sticks to the undercarriage and begins to clog the mower's blade. To keep the mower's engine from overheating, you must clean the undercarriage and remove the wet grass. Otherwise, the accumulation of the wet grass will make the engine work harder and eventually cause it to burn out.

This is what happens when you put too much food into your system. Fasting gives your body time to cleanse itself. Not allowing the body time to cleanse itself strains the digestive system and other organs. Why would you want to do that?

There are many types of fasts. For instance, there is:

- Intermittent fasting,
- Water fast,
- Bone broth fast,
- Green juice fast,
- Liquid nutrition fast, and
- A fasting mimicking diet, to mention just a few.

Because this can become a very confusing topic, this discussion is limited to intermittent fasting.

There is a difference between intermittent fasting (short periods of rest) and extended fasting (long periods of rest). An extended fast or long fasting lasts more than 36 hours whereas an intermittent fasting period is less. If you decide to do an extended fast, it **MUST** be under the supervision of a medical doctor or qualified health professional. Please, do **NOT** do an extended fast without proper medical supervision.

What happens to your body when you give your body time to rest between eating?

When you fast intermittently, insulin levels go down and glucagon goes up, which has been shown to have benefits such as increased metabolism, more energy, improved mood, and of course, weight-loss.

HOW AND WHEN DO YOU FAST?

Intermittent fasting is the practice of *not* eating food within a certain time period during the day. Intermittent fasts can last as little as four hours or as long as 36 hours.

For those of you who've never done intermittent fasting, begin with one of the most common approaches to intermittent fasting: avoid eating your meals within a 12-to-16-hour period each night.

Some research suggests that 16 hours is the optimal amount of time for creating the caloric restriction that happens during fasting and to give your cells time to cleanse themselves. However, other experts feel that 12 to 14 hours is sufficient to give your body time to cleanse itself.

Also, make certain you drink between eight and 16 ounces of water when you first wake up. This will help reduce morning hunger and prolong the fast and improve the cleansing process.

This is what an intermittent fast could look like: You finish dinner at 7:00 p.m. and you don't eat again until 7:00 a.m. That's it! That is a 12-hour intermittent fast.

This is really the easiest way to start any kind of fasting. You might already be implementing this without realizing it.

Be realistic about intermittent fasting. There will be times when you're going out with friends for dinner or attending other events that might be outside your period for eating. If this happens don't worry about it. You don't need to make a religion out of intermittent fasting. It is not a fixed rule. You don't need to do intermittent fasting every day. These are just guidelines to shift your hunger habit.

Experts have their own views and opinions about what is the best way to do intermittent fasting, whether it is 12, 13, 16, or 18 hours. You need to figure out and determine what is best for you. If you work the night shift or wake up at different hours, make your own fasting schedule.

The concept is that you're eating most of your food during a six-to-ten-hour period during the day and you're doing it when your body has adapted to the process. Go at your own pace. You don't want to force your body into an intermittent fasting regimen if it's not ready.

Don't force yourself into eating *only* during a six-to-ten-hour window of time if you're hungry the rest of the time. It means that intermittent fasting is not right for you at this moment. That doesn't mean you won't be able to do this in the future. Make small adjustments to your daily eating routine consistently over a long period of time until it becomes your habit.

Even though intermittent fasting has many benefits to help heal your body, it doesn't mean you can eat anything you want like processed foods and junk food, and it doesn't mean you can eat as much as you want. You still need to eat whole (holistic) foods and watch your portion sizes.

There are some people who should *not* fast. These include, but are not limited to, pregnant women, newborn babies, young children, high-level athletes who do intense training, individuals with a history of eating disorders, Type 1 diabetics, and individuals with pathological cachexia. (Cachexia is a condition that causes extreme weight-loss and muscle wasting. It is a symptom of many chronic conditions, such as cancer, chronic renal failure, HIV, and multiple sclerosis.)

HOW OFTEN SHOULD YOU EAT?

Contrary to popular belief, how often you eat does not matter much depending on each person's situation. If you eat the right types of foods, in the right portions, in the right environment and without distractions, then how often you eat becomes a matter of personal preference.

According to the International Society of Sports Nutrition (ISSN), "The preponderance of the research suggests that increased meal frequency does not play a significant role decreasing body weight/ weight composition." How often you eat doesn't appear to matter when calories and macronutrients are the same.

Another common misconception is that smaller, more frequent meals will boost your metabolism. Several research studies have examined the impact of how often a person eats—from 1 to 17 meals—on metabolic rate. The results show that it doesn't matter if you're a nibbler or a gorger. Of course, this assumes the food choices and amounts are the same.

It's your choice if you want to have smaller, more frequent meals throughout the day or eat one or two larger meals; just make sure the food quality and amount are the same. Overall, some people prefer intermittent fasting, some prefer time-restricted eating, and others prefer limiting food intake to one meal per day. My suggestions are you do *what works for you*.

Golden Rule Number Eight

Golden rule number eight is to think positive.

Your mindset matters. Without changing your mindset about health and a willingness to change your eating habits, any attempt to be healthy is futile.

Living a healthy lifestyle is hard.

Staying healthy, fit, and trim never stops. It's like running a marathon without a finish line.

Staying fat, overweight and eating unhealthily is easy.

Don't let other people tell you that you are unable to do something, and don't hold onto an assumption that you are unable to grow and learn from past failures. Legendary UCLA head basketball coach John Wooden said it best, *"Do not let what you cannot do interfere with what you can do."*

Our minds are the most important part of the body for overall health and wellness. Yet, it is the one area most weight-loss programs ignore or neglect because they want your repeat business. Your greatest enemy for reducing weight, shedding those unwanted pounds and your wellness lives between your ears. Your success in being begins when you change your mindset.

Your desire to be healthy is based on a combination of your thoughts, your feelings, and how those affect your eating habits and actions. This is your mindset. Your feelings lead to your emotions. Your emotions control your thoughts. Your thoughts control your actions. Your actions lead to your temperament. Your temperament determines your behavior, which predicts your results.

Mastering your behavior is paramount to your health and wellness success. And it all begins with your mindset. Have you wondered why it's so difficult to improve our eating habits? After all, we all know what to do, we just don't do it. Why is that?

It's not so much what we can do as it is what we will do.

The source of being unhealthy is poor eating habits based on poor choices.

So, why do you make poor choices?

Perhaps it's not so much the poor choices we make. Instead, it is our flawed relationship with food. It's from the way we think about food and our body.

Many people turn to food for comfort if they're having a bad day, are hurt, or upset. Do you? Have you thought, "I need some food to comfort me?"

In movies or TV shows, when someone is upset or hurt, the first thing they show is that person eating a pint of ice cream or stuffing cookies or cake into their mouth.

Many people enjoy food at social gatherings, holidays, and special occasions such as birthdays and anniversaries. *Rarely, if ever, do people think about food as fuel and nutrition for the body.* Perhaps we just don't care.

The obvious answer to improving our eating habits is to change our stinking thinking about food. Getting rid of the stinking thinking is easy to say, however, not so easy to do. Unfortunately, too many of us have negative thoughts that are non-supportive, and not just for being healthy—it applies to most everything else in life.

According to some research, 80 percent of our thoughts are negative and non-supportive.

Take a moment to contemplate what your life would be like if your thought process were reversed, and 80 percent of your thoughts were positive and supportive.

Negative thoughts are exhausting to the body. Further, complaining, whining, or diminishing your own self-worth also saps your energy by creating chemicals that weaken the body.

The good news is, if you can recognize a negative thought, you can consciously choose to change it. Instead of saying, "I can't lose weight," say, *"I have the power to control my weight. I have a strong urge to eat healthy foods and forgo processed foods."* The chemicals produced by your body as a response to this kind of thought are more likely to support you in fulfilling your goal.

The only way to override the negative and non-supportive thinking is with positive and supportive thoughts.

Use affirmations and visualizations as a tool to program your mind to believe and then take consistent and persistent action based on those thoughts.

Focus on what you can control and then go take some action based on those thoughts. Realize that your state of consciousness creates your reality, and your reality is yours to make whatever you so choose.

It's imperative that you create the thoughts you want about food and put them on autopilot, so they become second nature and natural. Do it to a point so that your thoughts are no longer negative but are positive. Your positive thinking becomes as normal as brushing your teeth.

If you don't learn to manage your way of thinking about food, you are doomed to a life based in failure and struggle with weight and health issues. Your old concepts about food will keep you stuck. T. Harv Eker said, "Consciousness is observing your thoughts and actions so that you can live from true decision-making in the present moment rather than being run by programming from the past."

Either you control your thoughts, or they control you. Either way, it's your choice. Training and managing your mindset are the most important skills you can learn in terms of both happiness and success. It's doable and you can do it.

Weight-loss programs tend to be a temporary solution because they're incomplete.

Most weight-loss programs don't help people change their thought process or their relationship with food. There is a lot of empirical evidence and data that proves the majority of those who lose weight fail to keep it off. They gain 100 percent of their weight back.

Again, if diets and weight-loss programs worked, the weight-loss and diet companies would be out of business.

Think positively. Watch your thoughts. Watch your words. They have an impact. You are not making a sacrifice by avoiding certain foods. You're making a choice. You are not depriving yourself of anything, i.e., sweets, ice cream, cookies, cakes, etc. You're making a choice. Remember, we all make choices. Think healthy.

Think in terms of releasing weight, rather than losing weight. Think in terms of reducing weight, not losing weight. When you lose something, you tend to want to find it. You are not foregoing that piece of pumpkin pie or pecan pie. You are making a choice not to indulge. Think "I'm Thinning!"

I'm not telling you that you can never enjoy a piece of cake or pie, or a scoop of ice cream. That is not realistic. If you do decide to indulge and enjoy some ice cream, cake, or pie, only have a small amount. Have a spoonful of ice cream instead of a scoop, or two. Have a sliver of cake or pie. You don't have to eat an entire piece. This can satisfy your craving and not set you back on your thinning journey. No one is perfect. If you do overindulge, don't beat yourself up over it. Just keep moving forward.

By the same token, don't keep making excuses for making exceptions. Exceptions tend to become the rule. I'm talking about those little voices in your head telling you, "It's OK to eat that candy bar or cookie," or "You've earned that piece of pie or dessert." No! It's not OK to have that candy bar or eat that cookie. No! It's not OK to "treat" yourself if you're still attempting to shed weight.

Do you want to reduce weight and improve your eating habits or not?

If so, what are you willing to improve and change to make it happen?

Can we agree that nothing about your weight and health will improve if you're not willing to do something different?

It may sound like you're getting conflicting information. You are right. The point you need to understand is, it's not OK to overindulge eating things you know aren't going to help you lose weight. Those chips you're thinking of having, don't. But every so often, if you do have some chips, it's not the end of the world. Just don't make it a new old habit.

Have you attempted to make healthy food choices only to have someone tell you, "Have just one, it won't kill you?" Or "One cookie won't hurt you." No, it won't hurt you. No, it won't kill you. However, it will prevent you from accomplishing your goal of getting rid of your extra weight. Be polite, but respectfully decline. Just say, "No, thank you." You do not need to give an explanation. Sometimes I'll tell someone, "It will look better on you than me." Or "More for you." Or "Better in the trash than on my ass."

There are many more variations of situations to make an exception so be wary. There will be those people who will tell you, "You can't lose weight, so just go ahead and eat." Or "You won't be able to do it. So, why bother?" Maybe it's your own little voices pelting you with negative thoughts. Or you've heard the statistic that 90 percent of those who start a diet fail. And of those who do succeed in dropping their pounds, 90 percent gain it all back. So, why bother?

Have you had those thoughts?

Don't believe them because they belong to those who can't. You can do it. Besides, **you are not dieting. You are changing your eating habits and lifestyle.** You are improving and changing your eating habits. You are among the 10 to 15 percent who can and will succeed in achieving a healthy weight and maintaining it. You are the exception because you are not participating in the new normal.

DECLARATIONS AND AFFIRMATIONS

Do you use declarations each day?

Do you use affirmations each day?

Declarations are different from affirmations. A declaration states the objective of doing something. Whereas an affirmation states that a goal is already happening. This might not be true for your weight-reduction, in which case, your mind will immediately dis- miss this statement.

Affirmation is basically just self-talk. It's a statement about ourselves or our situation that's phrased in the present tense as if the self-focused declaration is already true. We continually use affirmations subconsciously with words and thoughts and this flow of affirmations is what creates our life experience in every moment.

Behavioral psychologists have proven that more than 80 percent of our self-talk is negative. Have you said to yourself, "Positive declarations or affirmations won't work for me for eating healthy?"

That's a declaration itself. Just thinking of those words is a declaration. It also has negative consequences. Your perception of being unhealthy and overweight can cause you to gain weight or prevent you from dropping it. Researchers found that thinking of yourself as being overweight can turn into a self-fulfilling prophecy.

Declarations and affirmations are important for a healthy life because they work.

Unfortunately, most people engage in self-talk in a negative way. The types of affirmations people use are negative in nature. Do you use words and thoughts intended to build yourself up, or do you gravitate towards things keeping you down?

Have you thought, "Once I'm healthy and fit, I'll be good enough"? Or "I'm too fat and ugly now, but when I get fit and look better, I'll have a boyfriend."

This is negative motivation. While negative motivation can provide a short spurt of weight-loss drive, it will ultimately not work out in the long term. Negative motivation may help you lose 20 to 30 pounds, but you'll likely be mentally worse off than before, and you may even regain the weight you've lost.

To successfully have and maintain a healthy body, you'll need to fix the negative self-talk in which you've been engaging. The fix for this is simple. Here is how you can do it:

Identify the negative self-talk you've been using in your life. (It might help to write these down so that you don't forget them.)

Create positive affirmations around your negative self-talk. The goal here will be to literally "flip" your negative self-talk into positive affirmations.

Here are some examples:

- "I am not overweight" becomes "I am at my ideal weight."
- "I am losing weight" becomes "I am closer and closer to my ideal weight with each passing day."
- "I am not eating junk food or fast food" becomes "Everything I eat heals and nourishes my body which helps me reach my ideal weight."

Get control over your thoughts, over your words, and over yourself. It's going to require consistent work to reverse the psychological damage that negative self-talk causes within us. It won't happen overnight. However, give it enough time and the weight will melt off. More importantly, you'll have more energy, you'll feel better, look better, have sharper cognitive ability and mental alertness (no more afternoon brain fog) and improve your overall health.

It's important to use the present tense when you create your new positive affirmations because the present tense will make them feel more sincere, authentic, and genuine. This will accelerate your progress. If you use the future tense such as one day or someday, it puts it off. Make it happen now. "I am…"

If you find yourself thinking or engaging in any negative self-talk, stop yourself. Transform it into the positive, at once. Focus on what you do want, not on what you don't want, because what you focus on expands.

DAILY DECLARATIONS FOR A HEALTHY LIFESTYLE

Here are Daily Declarations for living a healthy lifestyle. These are my personal declarations. You can choose which ones you want to adopt as yours or you can create your own.

- I am in the process of being healthy, slim, and fit.
- I am strong and beautiful at my healthy weight.
- I eat proper portions. I enjoy using a salad plate instead of a dinner plate.
- I am an inspiration to others to live a healthy life. If I can do it, others can too.
- I am living a healthy lifestyle and improving each day.
- I am turning my body into a fat-burning machine.
- I am using creative alternatives to keep focused and committed to keeping my healthy living goals.
- I am accountable for my choices.
- I am resolved to sustain my reduced weight in a healthy manner.
- I am using positive words with myself and others.
- I am making food choices and decisions for my higher good regardless of what others might say or think.
- I am looking and feeling terrific. I love my body.
- I am letting my clothes tell me everything about being healthier.
- Even though I am not at my ideal weight, I love, accept, and appreciate my body.

"I AM GRATEFUL" STATEMENTS

Being grateful helps you feel more positive emotions, improves physical and mental health, reduces stress, promotes better sleep, and strengthens relationships. Below are some gratitude statements. These are my personal "I am grateful" statements. You can choose which ones you want to adopt as yours or you can create your own. Or you can continue to use your declarations because they are similar.

- I begin the day with gratitude. I am grateful for what I have and for what I shall receive.
- I am grateful, appreciative, and happy to be living a healthy lifestyle.
- I am grateful and happy to be healthy and fit.
- I am grateful to be strong and beautiful in my healthy body.
- I am grateful and happy to retain my healthy weight.
- I am grateful to be lighthearted.
- I am grateful for attracting joyful, sincere, loving relationships.
- I am grateful I eat proper portions. I enjoy using a salad plate instead of a dinner plate.
- I am grateful to be an inspiration to others. If I can do it, others can too!
- I am grateful to be living a healthy lifestyle and improving each day.
- I am grateful my body is a fat-burning machine.
- I am grateful to be accountable for my choices.
- I am grateful to use great alternatives to keep focused and committed to my goals.
- I am grateful to be resolved to sustaining my reduced weight in a healthy manner.
- I am grateful to use positive words with myself and others.

- I am grateful my healthy eating habits make me smile with pride.
- I am grateful to allow myself to make food choices and decisions for my higher good regardless of what others might say or think.
- I am grateful to look and feel terrific. I love my body.

To be successful with anything, you must be able to negotiate and communicate what it is you want. But sometimes the toughest sale of all is selling to yourself. It's like when you say to yourself, "I need to exercise today," another voice in your head says, "No, I'm too tired." So, then you say to yourself, "I'll do it tomorrow." Or "I'll do it after work."

Every person who has attempted to get healthy knows that battle. It's the self-talk, or management of it, that will get you through difficult times, or cause you to succumb. Don't let the negativity in, don't let your emotions even get started. Just tell yourself, "No thank you. I've practiced for this situation, and I can control myself."

Now you know what to do, and how to improve your eating behavior. The only question is… will you?

WHAT YOU FOCUS ON EXPANDS

Focus on what you want, because as Zig Ziglar, world-renowned salesperson and motivational speaker said, "When you focus on problems, you'll have more problems. When you focus on possibilities, you'll have more opportunities." With respect to being healthy, too many people focus more on their increased risk for type 2 diabetes, heart attack, stroke, cancer, and other ailments than on the solutions to their health issues. Did you know type 2 diabetes is preventable and reversable?

If you're focusing on the fact that you're unhealthy and living an unhealthy lifestyle, that is what life will keep serving you. In the health game, those who focus on the problem rather than the solution end up with more problems. According to Dagmar Fleming, *"The Power is in the journey to stay in the game — the game of life."*

People who successfully lose weight and keep it off focus on the solution. They believe in attaining their goal. They want it, and their actions are reflective of their belief. They look for ways to improve rather than reasons why they are unable. Focus on what you want to create rather than what you want to avoid.

It's imperative that you create the thoughts you want about food and put them on autopilot, so they become second nature and natural. Do it to a point that your thoughts are no longer negative, rather, they are positive. Your positive thinking becomes as normal as brushing your teeth.

"Positive Action Can Change Every Negative Situation."

– Darren Hardy,
New York Times best-selling author of *The Compound Effect*

Jan's Story

Let me tell you about my client, Jan. When Jan reached out to me, she was 63 years young. However, she felt old, tired, and depressed. She had been carrying around some extra weight for a few years. She had given up any hope of taking off those extra pounds. She believed that she was no longer capable of losing that weight. Jan thought she was old and that carrying extra weight was all part of being a senior citizen.

After a few weeks of being Jan's accountability partner, she told me, "I need an attitude adjustment."

"Why do you think you need an attitude adjustment?" I asked.

"Because we are the same age. And you are telling me about all your activities and trips you are doing. I'm getting ready to die."

I said, "You are right, you do need an attitude adjustment."

With my help and support Jan surpassed her goal to shed 30 pounds and ended up losing 45 pounds. Jan did the "I'm Thinning" process and told me she never felt deprived or hungry! She no longer feels like a senior citizen either. Jan said, "I feel young again." And, because of her new attitude, Jan met someone she is dating and is sharing a new life with.

Do you need an attitude adjustment like Jan?

Golden Rule Number Nine

WALK EVERY DAY

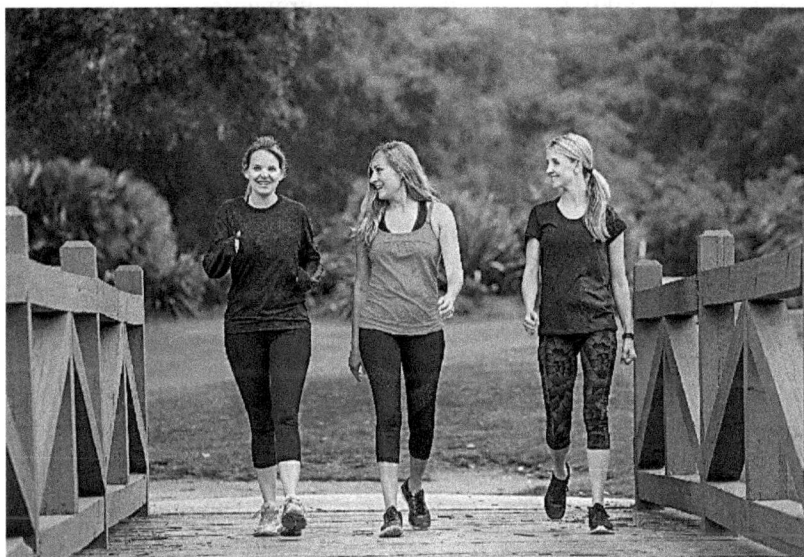

Golden rule number nine is to walk every day.

Walking is one of the most underrated exercises and physical activities you can do. Walking provides vast health benefits for everyone including weight-loss. Walking is for any person who is physically able to stand up and walk.

One of the biggest myths about health and fitness is the notion that you need to exercise for hours each day at the gym or health club to be fit. The truth is you don't need to go to a gym or health club to get fit because the best way for you to get fit is by walking…just walk thirty minutes to an hour each day. And, if you miss a day or two, don't beat yourself up.

Keep moving forward.

Actress Rebel Wilson shed 77 pounds by walking one hour each day. She told fans: "An Austrian doctor said 'Rebel, the best way for you to lose unwanted body fat is just simply walking. Doesn't have to be high intensity, doesn't have to be uphill, just moderate walking an hour a day. And if you can do that, for you, for your body type, it's like, the best way to lose unwanted body fat.'"

Actress Mindy Kaling, who reduced weight, also walks for exercise. During an interview with TODAY, Kaling said, "Sometimes I'll be like, well I have four different times today where I have 10 minutes so let's just walk instead of sitting down and checking Instagram. So instead of it being like one chunk of exercise in the beginning of the day or none at all, I'm now just deciding that I'm going to be a more active person all the time."

With a bit of planning, you can fit in an hour walk each morning before work or in the evening after work. Or, during a lunch break for one half hour. However, you do not need to do all your walking in one stretch of time. You can break it up into segments throughout the day depending on your schedule.

Walking doesn't require any special equipment. It's one of the easiest ways to become more physically active and it's a low-impact exercise. Some of the benefits of walking include:

- Reduces symptoms of depression and anxiety which could improve your mood.
- Reduces stress.
- Lowers low-density lipoprotein (LDL).
- Raises high-density lipoprotein (HDL) cholesterol (the "good" cholesterol).
- Lowers blood pressure.
- Reduces the risk of Type 2 diabetes and assists with the management of Type 2 diabetes.

- Reduces the risk for heart disease.
- Maintains strong bones and lean muscles.
- Builds aerobic fitness.

Best of all—you don't have to pay for it.

Walking can improve your health, promote wellbeing, and keep you active. Plus, it doesn't cost a thing. Despite what your fitness tracker says, you don't need to walk 10,000 steps each day to get the health and fitness benefits. Researchers suggest between 6,000 and 10,000, which is a more flexible target, making it easier to stick to.

However, you will not get buff or ripped just walking. If you want to do that you will need a trainer to be a guide for you and you will need to lift weights.

Before you begin any exercise program, please consult your physician or qualified health professional.

"If you are in a bad mood, go for a walk.
If you are still in a bad mood, go for another walk."

—Hippocrates

The Zorro Circle

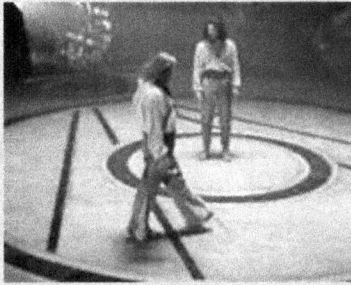

THE ZORRO CIRCLE

Limiting your focus to small manageable goals can expand your sphere of power

The Zorro Circle is a metaphor to limit your focus to master small, manageable goals, so later you can expand the scope of your ability and capability. In the movie *The Mask of Zorro*, Alejandro/ Zorro (played by Antonio Banderas) is a broken man. That is because as a young man, his ambition to fight villains and right the injustices in the world far exceeded his knowledge and skill set. After many attempts and many failures, Alejandro, frustrated, feels disillusioned and powerless. He surrenders to alcohol, falls into a deep despair, and loses his confidence.

Fortunately for Alejandro, he meets a mentor, Don Diego (played by Anthony Hopkins), an aging sword master. It is Don Diego who helps Alejandro regain his confidence by helping him gain a sense of control, giving him back his focus, conviction, and perseverance.

When Alejandro first started, he had no focus and no sense of control. He wants to do too much too quickly. However, he does not know where to start. This is how many people who want to get healthy and fit feel. They want to do too much too quickly. They are unaware of how to start to improve their eating habits. It can be daunting and overwhelming. Does this sound familiar?

There is a scene in the movie when Zorro's training commences. Don Diego places Alejandro in a small circle. Don Diego tells him, "This is called a training circle, a master's wheel. This circle will be your world, your whole life, until I tell you otherwise. There is nothing outside of it... As your skill with the sword improves, you will progress to a larger circle..."

The small circle is for Alejandro to control. A simple path to follow, he must master what is inside the circle before he can expand it or move on to the next circle. This is what you must do to improve and master your daily eating habits. You must master one circle [one rule] at a time. For instance, the first and most important daily eating habit you must master is to drink an adequate amount of pure water. This is the foundation of being healthy and living a healthy lifestyle.

Once Alejandro mastered control of that small circle, Don Diego slowly starts to expand his circle allowing him to attempt bigger and bigger feats, which one by one, Alenjadro achieves. Likewise, as you master drinking an adequate amount of pure water each day, then you can move on to the next circle, which is avoiding all processed and manufactured food products. And, once you master avoiding all processed and manufactured food products, then you move on to eating organic, whole, or holistic foods.

As Alejandro gained more confidence, he learned how to command his emotions and utilize his skills. None of Alejandro's achievements would have been possible had he not first been able to master that small circle. Similarly, what this means for you is it will be difficult, if not impossible, for you to achieve and maintain excellent health if you do not first master being able to drink an adequate amount of pure water and control your emotions.

If you forget the story,
Remember the lesson.

The Word "No" is a Complete Sentence

*"You must learn a new way to think
before you master a new way to eat."*

*– Karen Salmansohn,
Multi-best-selling author and award-winning designer*

There is a secret to achieving a healthy lifestyle without needing willpower. The answer is one word. That one word is "No."

The only way to win against your willpower, self-control, and discipline for living a healthy life is not to play. When you choose not to play, you win by default.

This is what I mean. If you're attempting to be healthier; willpower, self-control, and discipline will fail you 100 percent of the time. When confronted with certain situations on your health and wellness journey, you need rules.

In this day and age, to reduce weight in a healthy and sustainable manner you need insane focus to counteract the onslaught of the crazy distractions and temptations working against you. These factions and factors include TV ads for food and restaurants, other people in your life, social occasions, special events, and holidays. You must be focused and create sacred boundaries—rules.

WEDDING CAKE, CHEESEBURGERS, AND WINE

Special thanks to Darren Hardy, who provided the analogy of choices we make as it relates to rules and winning without willpower, self-control, or discipline when confronted with having a cheeseburger, wine, and wedding cake.

Let's say you're at a friend's home for an outdoor barbeque. Your friend is making the most delicious cheeseburgers with a special cheese. The buns are freshly baked, not the store-bought type. And he will be serving cheeseburgers with all your favorite condiments.

However, you're on a restricted diet to lose weight. What do you do?

Most people will succumb to the temptation to indulge in this special treat. Will you?

No, you won't because you're a vegetarian. You don't eat meat.

Your decision is made for you. You don't have a choice.

Okay, you're at the same get-together and your friend, being the gracious host that he is, offers you a glass of expensive wine. In fact, it's your favorite wine. What do you do?

Do you accept the gesture and drink the glass of wine?

No, you won't because you're three months pregnant. Most women know they are not supposed to drink alcoholic beverages during their pregnancy. Again, your decision is made. You don't have a choice because you don't drink. You respectfully decline. The decision is easy.

Here is another example. You're attending a wedding. The wedding cake is spectacular. A world-renowned pastry chef prepared it. People's mouths are watering because it tastes as delicious as it looks.

You, however, are watching your food intake because your mission is to eat healthily. What do you do?

Most people will take a bite or two of the cake just for a taste.

You, however, graciously decline to partake because you're deathly allergic to nuts. The wedding cake has nuts. Your choice is made for you because you don't eat anything with nuts. If you do, you'll have a severe allergic reaction that could cause death.

These examples are to prove two things to you about rules: you can resist when you must, and the only way to resist is if you must.

RULES:

A rule makes behavior decisions easy. Darren Hardy teaches don't say you "can't" do something. Turn a "can't" into a "don't." Change saying, "I can't have a glass of wine," "I can't have a piece of cake," "I can't eat the cheeseburger" to "I don't drink," "I don't eat wedding cake," "I don't eat beef."

The reason, according to Darren Hardy, is that "can't" can be negotiated with. Can't' means you're not in control and that you can be convinced to indulge.

Instead, say you "don't." "I don't drink," "I don't eat sweets as part of my daily food intake," or "I don't eat cheeseburgers while reducing weight." Using "don't" proves to those around you—as well as to yourself—that you are in control.

"Don't" also indicates that your statement is absolute. It's a rule. You follow rules all the time. You stop at red lights, you pay your taxes, you don't litter, etc. That's why establishing your own rules about eating will make it easier for you to succeed.

Systemize your own knowledge and create a set of eating rules for yourself. For example, you don't eat past 7:00 p.m. (or three hours before you go to sleep), you don't drink soda, diet soda, or fruit juices, because you only drink pure water, or whatever.

The rule standard is simple: under no circumstances will you answer anything but "No" or "No thank you," when offered something you know you shouldn't eat.

Just don't give in. Don't do it. Treat it like a pregnant woman does alcohol. For a pregnant woman, when offered alcohol, the answer should always be "No." Or take someone who has an allergy to food such as nuts. When asked if they will make an exception to eating a few nuts or products made with nuts, the answer for them is always "No." No matter what.

THINK OF "T.I.N.A."

T.I.N.A. is an acronym for the phrase, "There is no alternative." Think there is no alternative when making your decisions pertaining to the food you consume. Beware, however, of making exceptions because they tend to become the rule.

MAKE THE CHOICE ONCE

If you make the choice once not to indulge in eating refined sugar, processed food, cake, pie, doughnuts, ice cream, sweets, bread, snacks such as chips, crackers, or pretzels, then you never need to make it again. You'll reduce a thousand choices into one. The choice not to eat chips, pretzels, cookies, sweets, processed foods, etc. is yours because of the rule that you don't eat these things.

You'll avoid all those situational, conditional, "well, but" circumstances that collapse on you every time to challenge (and win over) your willpower, discipline, and self-control. You've already made the decision and the answer will be, "No, I don't indulge or partake eating…"

You eliminate the need to make a choice because the choice has already been made. It's a fixed rule of absolutely "No." No if 's, but's, or exceptions, and no need to re-think the decision every time in every circumstance and situation.

Steve Jobs, co-founder of Apple, Inc. said, "Focusing is about saying no." This can and should be your own mantra for wanting to be healthy and living a healthy lifestyle. Say "No" to convenience foods, i.e., frozen microwaveable meals, going through the drive-thru for fast foods, ordering pizza, or picking up a bucket of fried chicken.

Tip

If you want to stop eating unhealthy foods remove them completely from your home, car, office, and frequented living space.

Don't show up on an empty stomach to any social event, party, happy hour or outing where unhealthy food is going to be served. Eat before you attend.

The Psychology of Your Relationship with Food

By Michaela Gaffen Stone MS, BCBA,
Master Certified Nutrition Coach

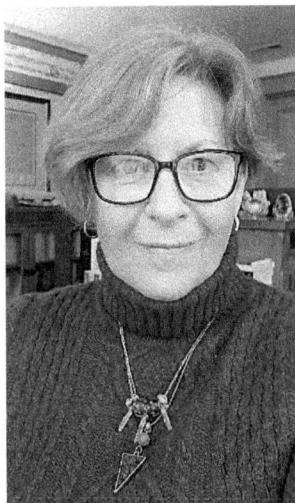

"Healthier Habits Healthier Life."
– David Medansky

To me, mindful, thoughtful eating is hugely important because without being fully aware throughout the entire eating process, you have no way of really understanding why you eat the foods you choose. There's some deep programming associated with the foods you choose to eat that you might not understand or be aware exists. Unfortunately, without exploring your relationship with food, any attempt to improve your eating habits and lifestyle will be brief and ultimately deeply disappointing. Subconsciously, you have a lot stacked up against you.

The food industry is selling products, not real food. The diet industry tends to push even more chemically laden products at you for more money with little to no benefit. The most important key element to understanding your relationship with food may have nothing to do with their manipulative and deceptive marketing and everything to do with the emotions you've attached to food.

For starters, why do you eat food? Is it for comfort? Does it help relieve stress? Is it for social reasons? Very few people understand that the true purpose of food is to provide nourishment for our bodies.

That's it. Plain and simple. Yet, many of us fail to understand this basic concept.

Missing Home

Let me tell you about a realization one of my clients had recently. She noticed she'd reach for certain pastries, not for their taste but because they reminded her of her home in Europe and her family there. It was like a little taste of home for her.

However, here's the kicker: she realized that the feeling of connection she craved was strongest when she thought about eating the pastry, not actually eating it. In reality, the pastry didn't satisfy her as much as she thought it would. It was all about her subconscious offering up pastries as a quick fix, without her even thinking about it.

Our brains are wired to take the easiest path, not necessarily the best one. It's like driving a familiar route without even thinking about the turns—you just do it automatically. And anything new or different is seen by our brains as a challenge, something to avoid.

That's what replacing one habit with another is like. The habit is—a loop that plays out without us even realizing it. The trick is to swap out those old habits for new ones, even if our subconscious fights us every step of the way. It's about making conscientious choices and decisions every day. The problem occurs because so often you are unaware that the habit is a habit because it is a routine behavior you no longer think about.

And you know what?

My client had her breakthrough because she thought about WHY she was eating pastries. She recognized the pastries did not provide her with the gratification she was seeking. It merely helped her to consume empty calories. Knowing her why allowed her to choose a different path. Instead of reaching for pastries, she decided to call her family. It was a simple change, which made a huge difference.

With that small change, she found real food freedom without relying on willpower. And for her, it's a game-changer.

So, what unhealthy food habits are you stuck in?

What do you reach for when you're feeling sad, stressed, or tired?

We all have our go-to comfort foods.

How much of that is a conscious choice, and how much is just automatic?

I Need Chocolate!

Here's another example based on my own experience. I remember the other day, I had this huge task hanging over my head, and by the time I finished it, all I could think about was chocolate. I didn't really need it. My brain, however, was screaming for it.

I went downstairs to tell my husband that I had finally completed the wretched task and with much more emphasis than I had known I was feeling said, "I NEED CHOCOLATE, NOW!!"

He immediately responded with the same level of intensity, "WE DON'T HAVE ANY!"

Luckily for me, my husband and I looked at each other and laughed. I ended up taking the dog for a walk instead.

What I learned from this experience is that I didn't really need chocolate. Rather, it was a subconscious program based on my emotional attachment to events long gone. That's why my husband and I both found it to be funny! We were all happier for it—especially the dog. He loves his walks.

The Doctor and Her Lunch

Another client of mine is an Emergency Room Doctor who told me the physicians lounge has food available, but it's not always good quality. The better items available predictably get taken first, and so she developed anxiety around being able to get food when she had a break - especially if her shift was busy and her break was late. She had not been aware of this worry gnawing away at her until she started reading the nutrition labels and searching for foods without additives.

Even then, the anxiety didn't reveal itself until she did some meal preparation at home and took food in with her. The realization that day came as a complete surprise to her. Bringing her own food had completely taken that anxiety away.

A Path Forward

The path forward for improving your eating habits and lifestyle *must* include food psychology. You need to delve deep inside your mind and thoughts. You must examine the tangled web woven by your thoughts and your emotions that lead to your eating routines, behaviors, and habits with food as the thread.

Think of the process as a plate of spaghetti. Each strand leads from a thought, emotion, or relationship to a particular food, or your wish to avoid an uncomfortable feeling. The problematic thought might hide under a lot of sauce; however, you're not aware of that underlying emotion.

By understanding the underlying psychological mechanisms driving your eating habits, you can choose to swap the pastry for a phone call, go for a walk instead of eating chocolate, or change worrying about not having enough food for lunch to knowing it's better to skip lunch than eat unhealthy food products. In other words, change what you are currently doing to develop a healthier and more thoughtful and mindful approach to food.

Are You Ready to Make Changes?

Here's an exercise for you to attempt at a meal or a snack. Don't worry, it won't hurt! The best way to discover possibilities is to do them, so let's explore:

- What do you think the food will taste like? How excited are you about it?
- Write down as much as you can about why you want to eat this, and what story you are telling yourself about the reasons to eat it? (Celebration? Do you "deserve" it? Comfort?)
- Bite #1 - is it as good as you thought it would be? Honestly. Is there anything about the food that is not what you expected? Write it all down!
- Bite #2 - how is this bite? As good? Not so much? Keep writing!
- Repeat step 2 until finished.
- How was it? Did it satisfy the reason you ate it? Was it as good as you thought?
- Finally, how do you feel 10, 20, 30 minutes later? How about a couple of hours later? Write it all down. Be as detailed as you can.

- Repeat this process with any food you feel you can't live without. There's some deep programming going on there, so let's uncover it!

Let me know how it goes.

You can email me at mikki@gaffenstone.com or find me on social media. If you need help, please reach out to me.

Bio

Michaela Gaffen Stone is a lifelong nomad and avid learner. She has lived in eight countries to date and has and continues to work in the health and wellness industry in most of them. In fact, she never met a time zone she couldn't work with. Michaela has gained deep insights into diverse cultures and their food practices along the way. As a Licensed, Board-Certified Behavior Analyst, Certified Wildfit Coach and Precision Nutrition Level 2 Master Coach, she specializes in boosting your natural immunity and overall wellness through attainable and sustainable gut health.

Facebook: https://www.facebook.com/michaela.stone.942
Instagram: https://www.instagram.com/mikkigaffenstone/
LinkedIn: https://www.linkedin.com/in/
mikki-gaffen-stone-15660a84/
Website: https://www.gaffenstone.com

Podcast:
https://www.inspiredchoicesnetwork.com/podcast/
navigating-complicated-relationships-with-mikki-gaffen-stone/

Author page on Amazon:

https://www.amazon.com/stores/Mikki-Gaffen-Stone/author/
B0CWDSLPGK?ref=sr_ntt_srch_lnk_1&qid=1710466314&
sr=1-1&isDramIntegrated=true&shoppingPortalEnabled=

The Pot Roast Story

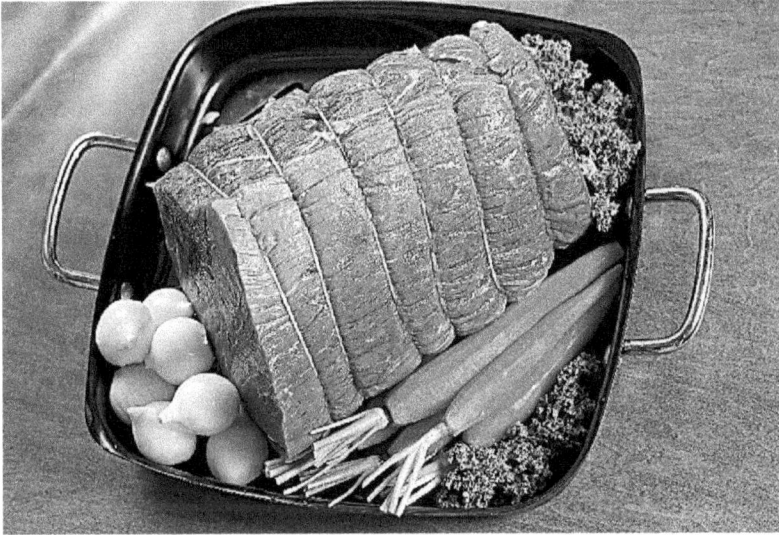

A young woman hosted a dinner party for her friends. She served a delicious pot roast. One of her friends enjoyed it so much that she asked for the recipe. The young woman wrote it down for her.

Upon reading over the recipe, her friend inquired, "Why do you cut both ends off the roast before it is put in the pan?" The young woman replied, "I don't know. I cut the ends off because I learned this recipe from my mom and that's how she has always done it."

Her friend's question got the young woman thinking. The next day she called her mom to ask her: "Mom, when you make the pot roast, why do you cut off the ends before you put it in the pan and season it?"

Her mom quickly replied, "Because that is how your grandma always did it and I learned the recipe from her."

The young woman became more curious. So, she called her grand-mother and asked her the same question: "Grandma, I sometimes make the pot roast recipe that I learned from mom which she learned from you. Why do you cut the ends off the roast before you prepare it?"

The grandmother thought for a while, because it had been a long time since she made the roast herself. After a moment she said, "I cut them off because when I was first married, the pan I had back then was too small. The roast was always bigger than the pan, so I had to cut the ends off to make it fit."

This is a great story since it teaches us that we do so many things without thinking about why we are doing them because that is how we were taught and how we have always done them. We rarely, if ever, question the reason or rationality of what we might eat or why we might prepare our meals a certain way.

This story demonstrates that before change can happen, you need to gain awareness of why you are doing what you are doing. For many of you, some of your eating behaviors were learned a long time ago because that is how your parents, grandparents, relatives, or friends ate.

An acquaintance of mine, John Canida, calls this "Dietary Duplication."

For your poor eating habits to improve and change, you first need to figure out or analyze why you like or dislike certain foods and beverages. If you drink soda or diet soda, ask yourself why. If you order certain toppings on your pizza, ask yourself why. Do you eat while watching TV, while driving, or at your desk while work-ing? If so, from whom did you learn this behavior? Maybe you are mimicking a fellow student, roommate, co-worker, or your parents.

Once you understand why you eat a certain way or what you eat, then change can begin.

John Wooden, legendary UCLA basketball coach said, *"When you improve a little each day, eventually big things occur. When you improve conditioning a little each day, eventually you have a big improvement in conditioning. Not tomorrow, not the next day, but eventually a big gain is made. Don't look for the big, quick improvement. Seek small improvement one day at a time. That's the only way it happens - and when it happens, it lasts."*

You did not gain all your weight in thirty days; you won't lose it all in thirty days. It takes consistency and time to be healthy and remain healthy.

The Nutrition Facts Label

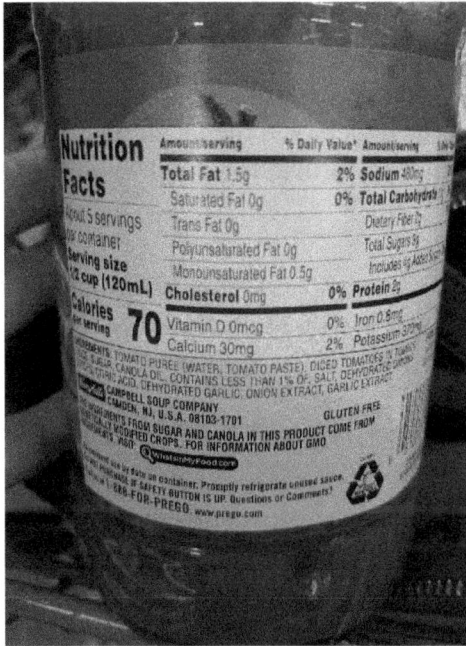

Capital One Financial promotes its credit card services by asking,

"What's in your wallet?"

William Devane in his commercials for Rosland Capital gold and silver asks, "What's in your safe?"

Perhaps the better question to ask yourself is, "What's in your food?"

Do you read the nutritional labels on the cans, packages, or boxes of the food you purchase?

If you do, do you understand what you're eating?

My guess is that you probably don't because most people won't.

Every packaged, or processed, product should have a label. (Note: some restaurants also have nutrition information available on their menus.) Nutrition Facts labels or Nutrition Facts panels communicate information about the food we eat. Data such as calorie count, amounts of sugar and fat, vitamin and mineral values, and ingredient contents help us understand the nutritional value of food products and make quick, informed buying decisions to meet a healthy diet.

The problem, however, is while that information might be interesting and somewhat useful, in my opinion, it is the fine print listing the ingredients that is most important.

READ THE INGREDIENTS!

Foods with more than one ingredient are required by law to list the ingredients on the label. Ingredients are listed by volume, with the higher amounts listed first.

Vani Hari (The Food Babe), New York Times best-selling author of *Feeding You Lies: How to Unravel the Food Industry's Playbook and Reclaim Your Health,* and other books, suggests you ask yourself these three questions before eating:

- What are the ingredients?
- Are the ingredients nutritious?
- Where do the ingredients come from?

If you are concerned about your intake of sugars, make sure that added sugars are not listed as one of the first few ingredients. Other names for added sugars include corn syrup, high-fructose corn syrup, fruit juice concentrate, maltose, dextrose, sucrose, honey, and maple syrup.

Let's look at a few Nutritional Fact labels from popular foods. For example, Prego Traditional Italian Sauce ingredients are tomato puree (water, tomato paste), diced tomatoes in tomato juice, sugar, canola oil. The label also states, "Contains bioengineered food ingredients. The ingredients from canola and sugar in this product are from genetically modified crops." In other words, they have adulterated the ingredients used to manufacture this product.

How about the ingredients in Cheerios Protein?

Notice how much sugar is listed as an ingredient (including corn syrup which is another sweetener.) And at the very bottom of the panel it states, "Produced with Genetic Engineering."

The front of the box is misleading and deceptive. Most people will look at the front and see "11g protein with milk" or "NO

ARTIFICIAL FLAVORS - NO COLORING FROM ARTIFICIAL SOURCES." And most people will believe this is a healthy choice. It is not.

Learn how to read the ingredients listed on the nutrition labels before deciding whether to eat the food or not. My best advice to you is to eat real food. An avocado or apple will provide you with more nutritional benefits than processed products.

A Matter of Perspective

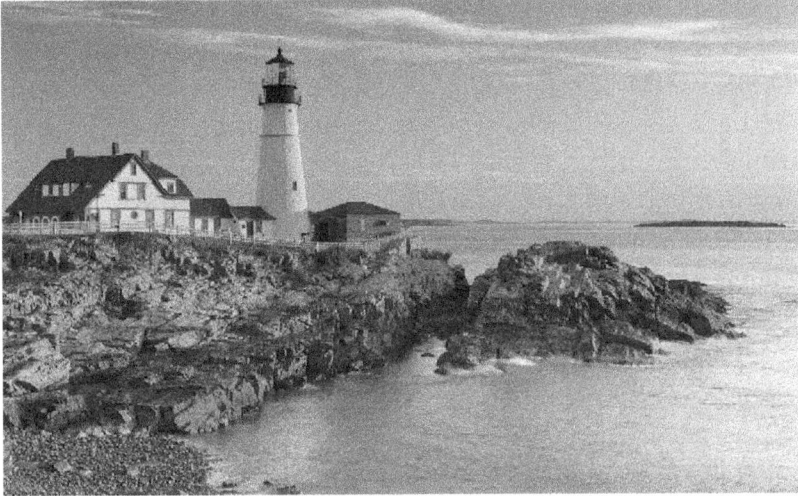

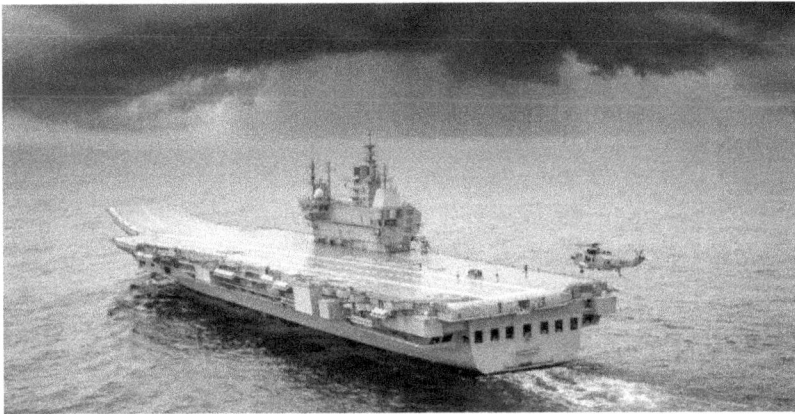

A U.S. Navy captain notices a light in the distance, on a collision course with his ship. He instructs a crew member to turn on the ship's signal lamp and send the message, "Change your course, 10 degrees west."

The light signals back, "Change yours 10 degrees west."

The crew member reports to the captain the response. The captain gets annoyed. He instructs the crew members to signal back, "This is the U.S. Navy. Our captain insists that you must change your course, sir."

The light signals back, "I am a Seaman First Class. You must change your course, sir."

Now the captain is angry. He instructs the crew member to signal, "I am an aircraft carrier. I am not changing my course."

The light signals back a final message, "I am a lighthouse, your call."

When it comes to your eating habits and lifestyle, are you acting similar to the U.S. Navy Captain who refuses to change course despite knowing the dangers and risks of doing so?

Consistency and Momentum

CONSISTENCY

Consistency is one of the important principles of your healthy life-style success. You can improve your health by changing your eating routines and food choices. Your improved eating routines and food choices become your new eating behaviors. Your new behaviors repeated become new habits. Eating habits compounded over time have a direct correlation to your health. Aristotle said, "We are what we repeatedly do."

Lack of consistency will derail you from realizing improved health. The start and stop process of diets kills the progress of your weight-loss pursuit and permanent results. Healthy and sustainable weight-loss success is about getting you to do what you know needs to be done consistently and permanently. After all, most of us know what to do to eat healthily. We just don't do it.

You can accomplish what seems incredible, extraordinary weight-loss results in short spurts. However, if your improved eating habits are not continued, eventually it is all for nothing. Perhaps that is why more than 90 percent of people who lose weight on a diet gain all of it back, some even more.

Moreover, consistency can work for you, or it can turn against you. Consider this: Many people would rather eat pizza every Saturday night for an entire year without thinking about the weight they are gaining. Then, they are shocked when they weigh 5, 10, or 15 pounds more than the previous year. However, if you consistently chose not to eat pizza every Saturday night, you might not gain those extra pounds.

Here is an example of why consistency is so important to achieving your optimal health.

Let's say that you've decided it is time for you to do something to be healthier and live a healthier lifestyle. You are going to change your eating habits. You are going to change your lifestyle. You are excited.

You declare to yourself and everyone what you are going to do.

You start with your new eating routines. You go for an entire week.

You get on the scale expecting to celebrate your new health journey. Except, the scale has not moved. Nothing. You haven't lost a pound. You look in the mirror and you don't see any change whatsoever. Your clothes still fit the same. This is when most people quit.

That is why most people who make a New Year's resolution to lose weight and get in better shape give up by late January. It is called discouragement. All your effort and no results.

This is when you need to have faith, to trust the process. The butterfly soars because it trusts the process of change. You unknowingly have started the compound effect. However, the results are too small and remain invisible for now.

Just keep eating healthy and making healthy food choices. Let's say you do this for another three to four weeks. Much to your horror, you have only shed a few pounds. Not like the television commercials that guarantee that you will lose up to 20 pounds in just one month. This is when other people really get frustrated – when, for example, after four weeks you have only shed a few pounds. You have said "No" to all the nachos. You have declined to eat all of the snacks, foregone all the candy bars, and resisted the cookies at the office or other places.

This is when another substantial percentage of people quit. And you might be in this place along your own health and weight-loss process. However, you keep the faith and trust the process. You remain consistent in your improved eating routines and behaviors. Now you start to see that your clothes are feeling a little looser, or you have more energy, more mental clarity, or just overall feel better. It is easier to keep consistent than it is to start over. If you slack off for even a few days or for a week because you went on vacation, or because of work deadlines, or the holidays, your old habits take over. All of the progress you have made is gone.

Don't believe me?

Why do you think more than 90 percent of people who lose weight on a diet gain it all back? Some gain even more than what they originally lost.

It is because they revert back to their old eating habits and poor food choices. It will take all that hard effort of seeing no results for a while just to get back to where you were. Will Smith, when asked what he did to get into shape for his roles in movies, said, "It is easier to stay in shape than it is to get in shape."

The average person will attempt 126 fad diets during their life-time. Albert Einstein said, "The definition of insanity is doing the same thing over and over and expecting different results." The definition of weight-loss insanity is attempting diet after diet and expecting different results. After all, diets are temporary and designed to fail. As I mentioned before, *if you want to lose weight and keep it off, don't go on a diet, change your diet.*

The big secret here is to continue with your improved eating rou-tines. Researchers in London found that it will take, on average, as long as 66 days to develop new habits. What is important to remember is that routines done consistently for an extended period of time turn into behaviors. Behaviors done consistently for an extended period of time turn into habits. This is one reason why old habits are so difficult to break and new habits are so hard to create. And that is the rub. It is difficult to maintain and keep those good healthy eating habits and so easy to return to bad unhealthy habits.

You need to master consistency, because if you remain consistent, it is easier to keep the weight off. We are an accumulation of what we do over time. However, we all drift. The difference between those who are able to keep the weight off and those who don't is the ones that keep it off adjust. They recalculate. Just as the pilot, or auto-pilot, in the airplane is always adjusting and recalculating its course.

MOMENTUM

Along with consistency is momentum. Momentum is powerful. Unfortunately, it is tragic if you lose your momentum. Think of a locomotive. It takes a massive amount of energy to get a train off a dead stop to move two inches forward. If you put a two-inch block in front of its wheels, no matter how much steam and energy you give it, the train will not move forward. It will remain blocked.

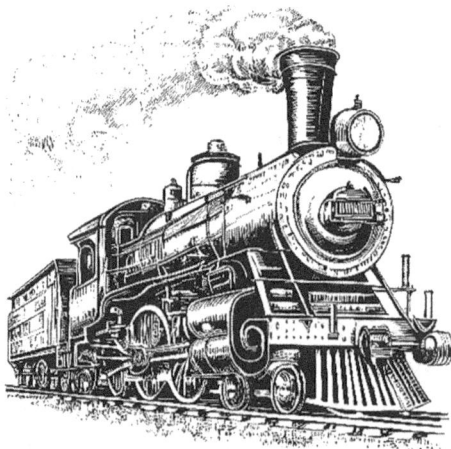

On the other hand, once you get that train moving and it settles into a consistent rhythm, it gets into that elusive force known as momentum. And once in that mode, it becomes nearly unstoppable. Instead of that two-inch block, you can set a concrete steel reinforced barrier on the track, and it will rip through it like crêpe paper.

A rocket ship blasting off into space requires a tremendous amount of thrust to overcome Earth's gravity. In order to escape the earth's gravitational pull, the rocket needs to produce 3.5 million kilograms (7.2 million pounds) of thrust to do so! As the fuel burns, the shuttle gets lighter, and less thrust is needed to push it up, so it speeds up!

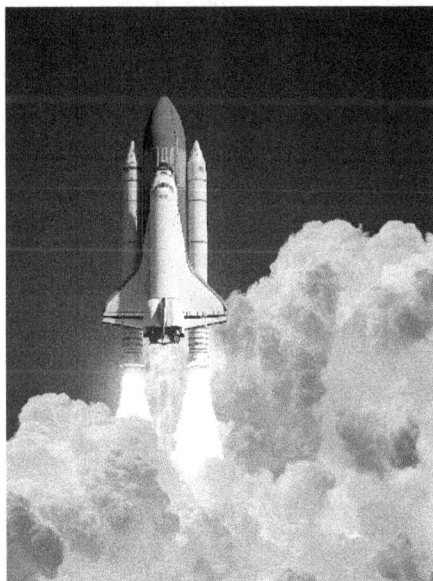

The takeaway here is that once you are in momentum on your improved health journey, it requires a lot less energy to keep moving in the right direction. This is where you want to get your daily eating routines, your patterns, behaviors, and habits – into momentum.

However, if you let your momentum dwindle, and your locomotive slows or comes to a complete halt (because you might have taken that two-week vacation, gotten busy at work, chose convenient processed and manufactured foods, ordered take-out or ate fast foods, for a while, especially around the holidays), it will require you to stoke that boiler once again with massive amounts of steam to get back to where you were. You are unable to afford to lose momentum. Once you get momentum, don't lose it.

So, how do you get and keep momentum?

According to Darren Hardy, "Momentum is created through the rhythm of systematized routines executed consistently." What this means for you is you need to have a system to achieve optimal health and a system to keep living a healthy life.

You want systems instead of goals. Losing 15, 20, 30, or more pounds is a goal. Learning to eat right is a system.

Having a goal is not going to help you to lose weight or get healthy.

The system to achieve the goal is what you want to focus your energy on. People tend to focus on their problem of being overweight instead of the solution to shed weight and improve their lifestyle.

Systems will always out do goals. Whatever your health goals may be, make sure you have a system to achieve them.

Then focus on the systems not the goals. In other words, focus on the process rather than the outcome. Outcomes are important. Of course, they are. However, if you become fixated on the outcome, it will work against you. That's because without focusing on the process, you will drift and get off track, making it harder to reach your weight-loss goal. Trust the process.

Make a lifestyle change instead of a life-changing transformation.

What does this mean?

People tend to get obsessed with making life changing transformations. Life-changing transformations usually fade away. Rather, get obsessed with the small daily lifestyle improvements that are needed to make the grand change possible.

Let me explain. Losing 50 pounds would be life-changing, right?

However, drinking 10 glasses of pure water every day is a new lifestyle. You want to concentrate on the lifestyle you need to have and maintain so you can attain the optimal health you seek.

> I no longer listen to what people say. I just watch what they do. Behavior never lies.
>
> - Winston Churchill

Two Wolves

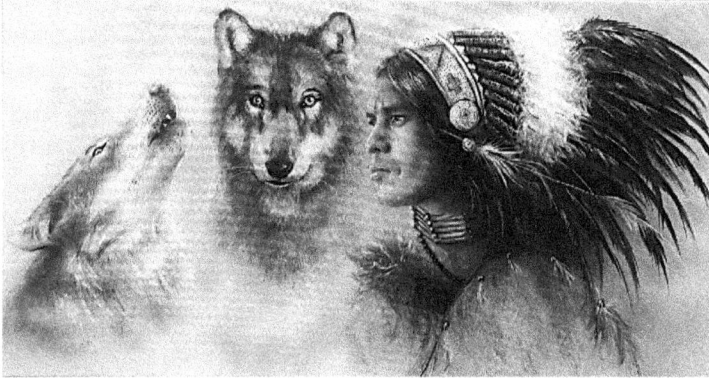

A Cherokee elder was teaching his young grandson about life.

"A fight is going on inside of me," he said to the boy. "It is a terrible fight, and it is between two wolves. One is evil. He is anger, envy, sorrow, regret, greed, arrogance. He is self-pity, guilt, resentment, inferiority, lies, false-pride, superiority, self-doubt, and ego.

"The other is good. He is joy, peace, love, hope, serenity, humility, kindness, benevolence, empathy, generosity, truth, compassion, and faith. "This same fight is going on inside of you and inside every other person, too."

The boy thought about it for a moment and then asked his grandfather, "Which wolf will win?"

The elder simply replied, "The one you feed."

When it comes to your health, eating habits, lifestyle, and food choices, which wolf is winning? Let's begin with the fundamental principles for excellent health so you can start to improve your eating and drinking habits to feed the "good" wolf.

One Last Message

If you find yourself struggling with your health journey, take some time to reflect and answer the questions below. Write out your answers either in your food journal or on a piece of paper. You might find your solution in doing self-reflection.

What Existing Eating Habits or Behaviors Do You Need to Expand?

For example,

- Can you drink more pure water?
- Can you eat more dietary fiber?
- Can you eat more vegetables?
- Can you eliminate processed and manufactured foods?

What poor eating habits or behaviors do you need to improve or stop?

For example,

- Can you stop drinking soda or diet soda?
- Can you stop going to the drive-thru, ordering pizza, picking up a bucket of fried chicken, or eating frozen microwaveable foods?
- Can you stop using ketchup as a condiment?
- Can you take more time to eat your meals instead of eating them while working or watching TV?
- Can you stop eating at least three hours before you go to sleep?

What new eating habits or behaviors do you need to start?

- For example,
- Can you start using a salad plate instead of a dinner plate?
- Can you eat slower?
- Can you start drinking pure water?
- Can you start using a salad plate instead of a dinner plate to control your portions?

What are your top three modifications or improvements to your daily eating routine and how will you implement them?

1. _____
2. _____
3. _____

TOUGH LOVE QUESTIONS TO ASK YOURSELF

- STEP 1: Affirm your health goal, i.e., reducing A1C, reducing cholesterol levels without taking statins or other types of drugs, reducing weight, etc.
- STEP 2: Ask yourself if you think you are on or off track.
    o Are you on or off track to hitting your goal?
    o Follow-up question:
    o If you are on track, what makes you feel that you are on track?
    o If you are off track, what do you need to do to get back on track?
- STEP 3: When you self-confess, ask yourself:
    o "Why do you think that is?"
    o Why do you think you are off track with your weight-loss plan?

YOU CAN DO IT – START NOW!

Learn From Your Past Mistakes

Based on Darren Hardy' Darren Daily

August 22, 2023

There's a story about two elk hunters who were flown into a remote valley in Alaska. By the end of the hunt, they had four elk to bring home.

When their pilot returned to take them out of the valley the pilot saw the four elk and said, "Here's a problem. The plane can only carry two elk."

The hunters were outraged. They said, "We were here just last year. The plane that carried us out was the same. The weather was the same and we had four elk then too."

The pilot said, "Well okay. I guess you guys know best then."

So, they loaded up the plane with the hunters and the four elk. The plane took off. As the plane started climbing out of the valley, it started to struggle. It began to lose altitude. The engine sputtered and gave out. The plane crashed.

As the hunters stumbled from the wreckage, one hunter asked the other, "Do you know where we are?"

The other hunter replied, "I don't know for sure, but I think it's a mile from where we crashed last year."

To err is human. However, why do some people make the same errors over and over again?

Do you procrastinate about improving your eating habits and lifestyle over and over again?

Do you continue to eat too much highly processed, manufactured, and convenience foods?

Get this, the largest underlying cause of death in America is related to the food and beverages we consume. Heart disease is the leading cause of death for both men and women. This is the case in the U.S. and worldwide. According to the Center for Disease Control (CDC) Leading Causes of Death are:

- Heart disease: 695,547
- Cancer: 605,213
- COVID-19: 416,893
- Accidents (unintentional injuries): 224,935
- Stroke (cerebrovascular diseases): 162,890
- Chronic lower respiratory diseases: 142,342
- Alzheimer's disease: 119,399
- Diabetes: 103,294

It seems our brains don't learn from past mistakes as much as we might hope.

Educating people on poor eating choices and habits of the past does not prevent them from doing it over and over again. How often have you told yourself you'll enjoy the donut today and start watching what you eat tomorrow?

When you give in to your urges you feel like a failure, which only makes you feel guilty and only encourages you to make more mistakes.

We are all capable of making the same mistakes over and over because under stress we tend to retreat into habits of emotion that are regulated and formed by toddlerhood. This is what neuroscientist Danie Levitin calls "Toddler Brain."

Darren Hardy explains that the toddler brain is what we resort to when we get stressed or overtaxed from physical or mental exhaustion. And due to today's advances of technology, information overload, and overstimulation today's environment has caused our lives to be dramatically more complex than our brains have evolved to be able to handle. This causes the human brain to retreat more and more into the toddler brain resulting in impulsiveness, poor judgment, and the inability to think through the consequences of that behavior. That's why you reach for that snickers bar or other candy bar for comfort.

So, what can you do to prevent toddler brain from taking over?

Get your 7 to 8 hours of quality sleep, exercise or be physically active, eat healthy foods, meditate, or have quiet time. Focus forward. Stop dwelling and lamenting about the past mistakes you made. Learn from those mistakes. Otherwise, you'll be doomed to repeat them. Focus on what you want to accomplish and view it from a fresh angle.

Benefits of Apple Cider Vinegar for a Healthy Life

Apple cider vinegar, ("ACV"), is a vinegar made from apple cider that has been fermented. Paul Bragg, N.D. Ph.D. described apple cider vinegar as "Nature's most perfect food." It contains acetic acid and lactic acid, as well as beneficial bacteria.

Apple cider vinegar has been around for thousands of years and used in a variety of health treatments and therapies. Roman soldiers drank "posca," apple vinegar with spices, as a stimulating, invigorating and fortifying drink. Hippocrates, the father of Western medicine, was already using vinegar as an antiseptic for coughs and colds as far back as 2500 years ago. And he also mixed vinegar with honey as a general tonic for good health.

Apple cider vinegar has many health benefits. These include:

- Helps the body reduce fat
- Improves digestion
- Balances pH levels
- Helps to maintain blood sugar levels
- Promotes detoxification of liver
- Increases metabolism
- Suppresses the appetite
- Helps in oxidation of stored fat
- Contains pectin, a naturally occurring soluble fiber
- Is rich in calcium and potassium – which promote weight loss

What is important to remember is it will only provide results if used consistently over a prolonged time. Be patient.

NOTE: Never drink undiluted apple cider vinegar. Apple cider vinegar should be consumed in water or another liquid because the acid can ruin tooth enamel.

Apple cider vinegar can be used as a salad dressing by mixing 1/2 to 1 teaspoon with 1 tablespoon of extra virgin olive oil and 1 to 2 tablespoons of lemon juice. (Maybe add some ground black pepper and garlic.)

Benefits of Lemon for a Healthy Life

Lemons are a nutritious fruit that might provide you with several health benefits. The benefits of freshly squeezed lemon juice include:

- Promotes hydration
- Good source of vitamin C
- Supports weight loss
- Aids digestion
- Prevents kidney stones
- Lowers the risk of stroke
- Lowers blood pressure

Simply mix one tablespoon of apple cider vinegar and one tablespoon of lemon juice in eight ounces of pure water and drink it in the morning.

Food Journal

The most common reason people keep a journal is for weight loss. However, a food journal is an excellent method to improve your eating habits. The four most common obstacles to keeping a food diary are:

- People are embarrassed or ashamed about what they eat.
- People have a sense of hopelessness, a feeling that it won't help to fill out a food diary.
- People feel it's too inconvenient to write down what they eat and drink.
- People feel bad or get upset with themselves when they "slip up."

A journal, however, is an effective tool to improve your overall health and wellness because it's been proven that keeping track of what you eat, and drink is the most effective method for controlling and changing your daily eating routines, behaviors, and habits. Whether you call it a daily food diary, diet journal, calorie tracker, food journal, or diet log, keeping track of your food intake is all about accountability.

It's not what you do when someone is watching, it's what you do when no one is watching. Be honest with yourself. Keep your integrity. Tell the truth. Record in your log if you indulged and ate the slice of birthday cake at the office party. No one is judging you.

In 2009, a group of researchers funded by the National Institute of Health published a study for a different approach to losing weight. They asked 1,600 participants to write down everything they ate for at least one day per week. Notice I said one day per week, not every day.

After six months, those who kept a food log lost twice as much weight as those who didn't. The researchers learned that many participants started looking at their entries and finding patterns they didn't know existed.

The participants started to implement different behavior modifications that were not suggested by the researchers. Some participants noticed they snacked at 10:00 a.m. so they started keeping an apple or banana in their desk for a midmorning snack instead of hitting the vending machine. Others started using their journals to plan future meals, such as dinner, so they could eat healthier rather than stop at the drive-thru for fast food or junk food in the fridge.

According to a study by Kaiser Permanente's Center for Health Research in 2008, keeping a food diary can double a person's weight loss. Their findings were published in the August 2008 issue (Volume 35, Issue 2, Pages 118–126) of American Journal of Preventive Medicine. Jack Hollis Ph.D., a researcher at Kaiser Permanente's Center for Health Research, said, "The more food records people kept, the more weight they lost. Those who kept daily food records lost twice as much weight as those who kept no records. It seems that the simple act of writing down what you eat encourages people to consume fewer calories."

The Kaiser Permanente's study was conducted in four cities, Portland, Oregon; Baltimore, Maryland; Durham, North Carolina; and Baton Rouge, Louisiana. In involved 1,685 middle-aged men and women over six months. The average age of the participants in the study was 55. Food journaling isn't easy or convenient, however, done consistently, it can help you move to more healthful choices. It allows you to keep track of all aspects of your dietary behaviors and habits.

You need to do the *Every Day Health Choices - 9 Simple Golden Rules to Live a Healthy Life* because knowledge without using it is a waste.

The Daily Journal will help you track what you are eating. However, below are 15 actions you can choose from to do to begin to build and form new eating habits and a healthy lifestyle.

Drink a minimum of 64 ounces, or one-half of your total body weight in ounces (if you weigh 200 pounds drink 100 ounces) of pure water.

- Eliminate foods with added sugar, i.e., candy bars, cookies, cakes, pies, pastries, cereals, ketchup, etc. Added sugar is "Kryptonite" when you're losing weight, not to mention your overall health. Cut it out and watch the pounds fly off.
- Avoid drinking soda and/or diet soda. Cutting out all soda for a month can drastically help you lose weight and improve your overall health.
- Eliminate all condiments, i.e., ketchup, mayonnaise, relish, etc. – Condiments have calories, too! Eliminating them and enjoying the taste of your healthy meal will shave calories and shed pounds.
- Eliminate white bread and pasta. Most breads and pastas are just no good, and you might be surprised at how many simple carbohydrates and calories they contain. If you can't remove them entirely, do your best to swap them out for Ezekiel Bread (found in the frozen section) instead.
- Eat mostly organic, or whole, holistic foods, i.e., vegetables, fruits, legumes, raw nuts, berries, beans, grass-fed beef, wild caught fish, and free-range chicken.
- Take at least 10 minutes to eat breakfast, 30 minutes to eat lunch and 30 minutes to eat dinner.
- Avoid eating while working at your desk, while on the computer, while driving, and while watching TV.
- Avoid eating dessert for 30 days – Hey, no one said this would be easy!!!

- Eliminate adding milk/sugar in your coffee or tea. Milk and sugar might taste nice, but they have extra calories. Cutting them out can help you improve your overall health.
- Walk 30 minutes to an hour each day. It does not need to be done at one time. You can break up your walks into 10- or 15-minute segments throughout the day.
- Eliminate alcohol. – Alcohol has calories. It also lowers inhibitions and can lead to over-eating. Let's not forget that hangovers also make exercise unappealing. Staying alcohol free for a month might be just what you need to jump start your weight loss. If you are unable to stop drinking alcohol for 30 days, you might have bigger issues to resolve.
- Eliminate fast food. Fast food is calorie-dense. Substituting it for healthier meals can significantly reduce calorie intake and promote general health and wellness.
- Give your body time to digest and process the food you consume by not eating for 12 to 14 hours at night (if you stop eating at 7 p.m. your first meal should be at 7 a.m. or later. Preferably later.) You should also drink 16 ounces of water first thing in the morning. This will help hydrate you and reduce your appetite.
- Get a minimum of seven to eight hours of quality sleep each night.

The Woman and Her Missing Keys

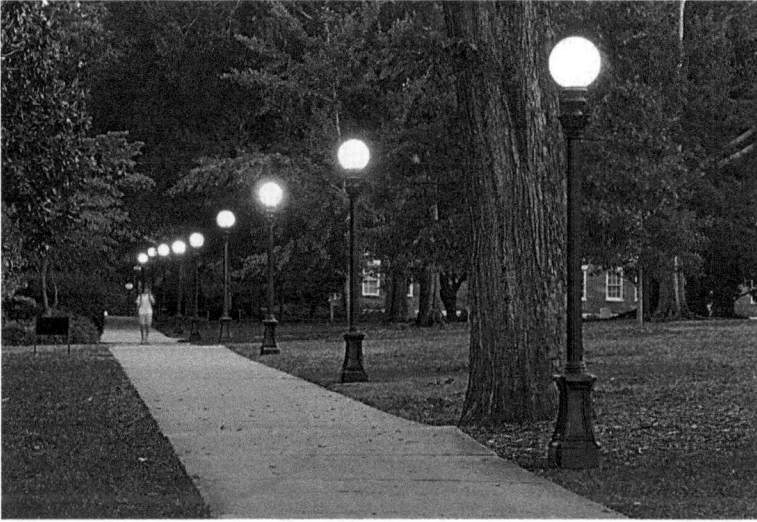

There is a story about an elderly woman who went for an after-dinner walk. While on her walk she dropped her keys. She kneeled down on the sidewalk under a streetlight and began searching for the missing keys.

Several neighbors and other people passing by offered to help. After five minutes none of them could find the keys. Finally, one passerby asked, "Lady, where exactly did you drop your keys? We've covered every inch around here!"

The woman pointed to an area in the darkness about five feet away.

"Then why in the world are we looking over here?" the passerby asked.

The lady replied, "Because the light is so much better here!"

This story explains why people are overweight and fail to live a healthy life and lifestyle.

Diets and health habits are like the streetlight to the woman because like the woman, fat and overweight people are looking for solutions where the light is brightest. People love to believe they can lose weight on the latest trendy diet or instantaneously get healthy with a magical supplement. I am here to tell you there are no shortcuts to becoming healthy and staying healthy. There is no miraculous fruit, berry, nut, vegetable, or supplement to permanently lose weight. It does not exist. If there was, we'd all be thinner.

There is no lotion to rub on your belly to get rid of fat.

There is no genie in a bottle to grant your wish of being thinner and healthier.

Two Frogs and the Pit

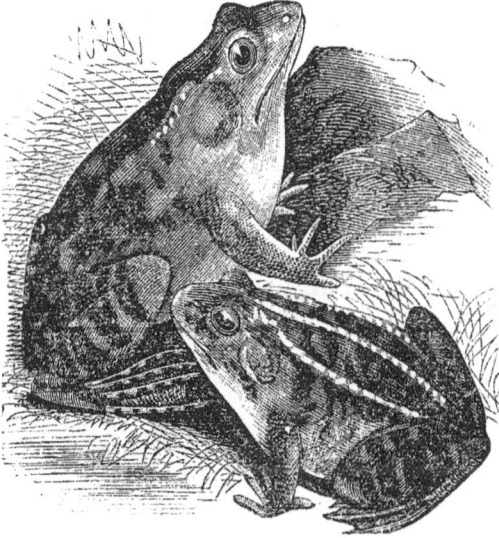

Several frogs were hopping through the forest when two of them accidentally hopped into a deep pit. The other frogs stood around the pit, and, seeing how deep it was, they told the two frogs that they couldn't help them. There was no hope. They were doomed.

However, fighting for their lives, the two frogs ignored the others and started jumping to get out of the pit.

The frogs at the top continued to tell the frogs in the pit to give up, as there was no way they would be able to jump out.

After jumping as high as they could over and over, one of the frogs listened to the others and gave up. He accepted the fate of his death.

However, the other frog continued to jump with all of his might. The crowd of frogs yelled down the pit for the frog to just stop. He wouldn't make it.

The frog ignored their warning and jumped even harder. The frog persisted until he finally got out. Upon reaching the top, the other frogs said, "We thought there was no way any frog could jump that high, couldn't you hear us?"

The frog then signaled to the others that he was deaf, and he thought that the frogs standing around the pit were encouraging and cheering him on the whole time. The lesson of this story is that when it comes to your health success, the words of others can greatly impact your attitude and actions. Ignore the naysayers. Only engage with those who encourage and believe in your ability to succeed. Think about what you say to people before speaking so you can make sure what you're saying is supportive. Your support (or lack thereof) could make the difference between success and failure.

Airplane Off Course

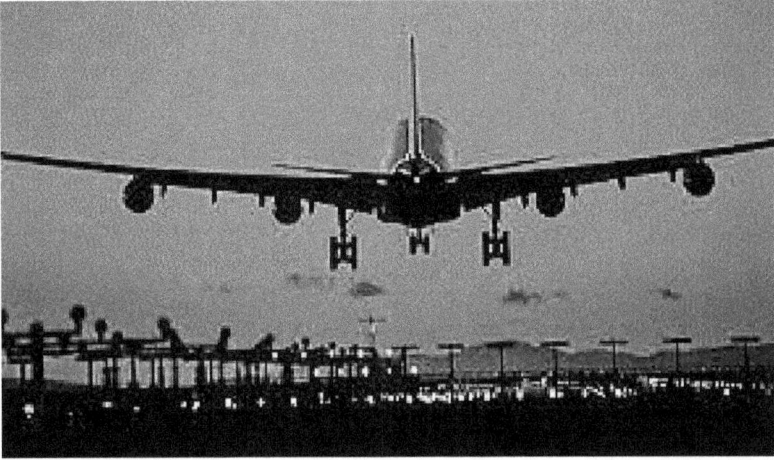

To achieve your optimal health goals, you must do as a pilot of an aircraft does. That is, you must be prepared to make continual course corrections.

An airplane traveling from Los Angeles to New York will end up hundreds of miles from its intended destination by being pointed merely one degree off course at the beginning of the flight. However, the average plane traveling from LA to New York will be off course more than 90 percent of the time along its journey. Each time the plane drifts slightly off course, its computerized gyroscope corrects it. The gyroscope recalibrates and corrects the flight path to hold the nose of the plane directly toward its destination.

On your health journey, you will also be off track much of the time. That is because old habits are hard to break, and new habits are difficult to create. What is important to remember is the key to living a healthy lifestyle is to keep correcting your eating behaviors to put you back on track. None of us is

perfect. We all make mistakes. Those who succeed learn from their mistakes to improve and get back on course. Those who do not succeed in attaining their best possible health fail to keep correcting their eating behaviors and lifestyle

The Benefits of a Corporate Health and Wellness Program

*Special thanks to John D. Allen
and Dr. Dennis Cummins for inspiring this chapter.*

In today's competitive corporate environment, offering a result-oriented employee health and wellness program is an imperative strategy for businesses aiming to thrive. Implementing the right corporate health and wellness program offers numerous benefits to employers, translating into reduced absenteeism, enhanced employee retention, boosted morale, improved productivity, and significant cost savings on healthcare costs. This chapter explores the underlying importance of investing in employee well-being for enhanced corporate profitability and overall success.

REDUCING EMPLOYEE STRESS AND BURNOUT

What is your company's biggest problem when it comes to your employees as it relates to their health?

For most corporations, it is employee stress and burnout.

Employee stress and burnout have become prevalent in today's workplaces, leading to sizeable adversity on both individual well-being, organizational performance, and profits. According to Forbes, corporate burnout in the U.S. alone costs $1.8 **TRILLION** in lost productivity each year.

High levels of stress can result in burnout. Burned-out employees tend to be less focused, more likely to make mistakes, and take longer to complete tasks. This can lead to lower productivity, which can cost a company money thereby lowering profitability. Burnout can also cause other issues that are detrimental to an organization's profits and revenue, including:

- Increased absenteeism. Employee time off often requires an organization paying for paid leaves, temporary replacements, or overtime.
- Higher turnover rates because burned-out employees often look for a different job.
- Damage to company culture because burnout causes a toxic work environment that leads to lower morale.
- Increased health care costs because chronic exhaustion, anxiety, depression, and other stress-related disorders, which can increase medical appointments, prescriptions, and treatment expenditures are a direct result of stress and burnout.

In other words, employee stress and burnout have a direct major adverse effect on an organization's bottom line.

A corporate health and wellness program can be instrumental in mitigating these issues and cultivating a healthier, more resilient workforce. By addressing the root causes of stress and burnout through comprehensive wellness programs, employers can create a healthier, more engaged, and more productive workforce. Reducing stress and preventing burnout not only improves employees' quality of life but also enhances their performance and commitment to the organization, ultimately benefiting the company's profitability and sustainability.

REDUCED ABSENTEEISM AND ENHANCED PRODUCTIVITY

It's a fact that when staff members are out for any extended periods of time, it costs the company money – just how much might surprise you. In the U.S. absenteeism costs employers $3,600 per hourly employee per year. That's a lot of money diverted from net profits.

One of the most immediate and measurable benefits of a corporate health and wellness program is the reduction of absenteeism and enhanced employee productivity. When employees are healthy, both physically and mentally, they are more likely to be engaged, focused, and efficient in their work. Chronic health conditions, stress, and poor lifestyle choices can lead to frequent sick days, decreased energy levels, and lower overall productivity.

A well-structured health and wellness program addresses these issues by promoting healthy habits such as proper hydration, regular physical activity, balanced nutrition, stress management, and preventive care. For example, regular physical activity has also been linked to improved mental health, leading to better concentration and reduced feelings of anxiety and depression.

Moreover, health programs that include mental health support, such as mindfulness training and stress management, can significantly reduce the impact of mental health issues as it relates to productivity and improve morale. Employees who feel supported in their overall health endeavors are more likely to maintain high performance levels and less likely to take extended leave due to illness, burnout, or mental health crises.

The cumulative effect of these health and wellness initiatives is a workforce that experiences fewer sick days and exhibits higher levels of productivity. This boost in productivity directly contributes to the company's bottom line by increasing output and operational efficiency.

REDUCED EMPLOYEE TURNOVER
AND INCREASED MORALE

Perhaps your biggest problem when it comes to employee health is employee retention.

High employee turnover and low morale significantly impacts the bottom line for many organizations because of the increased recruitment and training costs as well as disrupting team cohesion and productivity.

How much does it cost your company to train a new employee and how does high turnover effect profits?

According to the Work Institute's 2020 Retention Report, on average, depending on the position to be filled, *it can cost a company between one-half and one and two times the annual salary for the position to be filled*. A corporate health and wellness program can play a pivotal role in addressing these issues by fostering a positive work environment and demonstrating a commitment to employee well-being. In other words, it shows that your company cares about its members.

Employees are more likely to stay with an organization that values their health and provides resources to support their overall well-being. Health and wellness programs that offer benefits such as health screenings, nutrition coaching, fitness classes, stress reduction resources, and meal planning send a clear message that the employer cares about the holistic well-being of its staff. This sense of being valued and supported can significantly boost employee morale, job satisfaction, and team members are more likely to remain loyal to the company.

A positive work environment where employees feel supported and valued leads to higher engagement levels, better teamwork, and a more cohesive organizational culture. This increases employee retention thereby reducing turnover rates and can also enhance the company's reputation as an employer of choice, making it easier to attract top talent.

COST SAVINGS ON HEALTHCARE COSTS

The financial implications of employee health are significant, with rising healthcare costs being a major concern for employers. Poor employee health, particularly due to chronic conditions and lifestyle-related diseases, leads to higher medical claims and increased health insurance premiums. By investing in a comprehensive health and wellness program, employers can mitigate these costs and achieve substantial savings. Further, health insurance providers may offer a price break for having an employee health and wellness program.

Consider this; 60 percent of employees are overweight, 40 percent are either type 2 diabetic or pre-diabetic, 28 percent have Metabolic Syndrome, and 80 percent have regular high-impact stress.

So, what does mean for you?

Employee diabetics cost $15,000 more than a non-diabetic. Obesity and related issues are estimated to cost $9,000 in direct and productivity costs. It is estimated that 75 percent of all health care costs come from *preventable* and r*eversable* lifestyle diseases.

The return on investment (ROI) for health and wellness programs is well-documented. A study by RAND Corporation indicated that for every $1invested in a health and wellness program resulted in approximately $1.5 in lower healthcare costs. Other studies have shown that for every dollar invested in wellness programs, employers can expect to save several dollars in healthcare costs. Harvard researchers that conducted 26 studies on wellness programs found that for every dollar spent on a health and wellness program there was a $3.27 reduction in medical costs and $2.73 drop in absenteeism costs.

A methodical review of 56 published studies of corporate health programs showed that result based workplace health programs can lead to 25 percent savings directly correlated to each area, including, however not limited to, absenteeism, health care costs, workers' compensation, and disability management claims costs. These savings can be reinvested into the business, enhancing overall financial performance and sustainability.

Lifestyle interventions, such as weight management initiatives, physical activity programs, and nutrition counseling, can also lead to significant cost savings. For instance, employees who maintain a healthy weight are less likely to develop *preventable* chronic conditions such as hypertension, diabetes, and heart disease. This reduction in chronic disease prevalence translates into lower healthcare costs for both the employer and the employees.

The benefits of implementing a result focused corporate health and wellness program extend far beyond improving employee health because it can create a healthier, more productive, and more engaged workplace, ultimately leading to increased profitability.

What does all this mean to you, the CEO, President, or Owner? It means priceless goodwill for the company because people feel valued. When people feel valued, they are happier and work harder. Employees are more productive because they take pride in their work, they take ownership of the job they do for the company. Employees feel they are part of the team and not just a number. These are all things that keep employees happy, content and not looking to go elsewhere. That's what it means when a company cares about its employees.

Thank You

Thank you for investing in yourself and in this book. If you have found value in this book, if it has helped you in any way, please leave an honest review. In addition, please consider giving a copy to five people whom you care about and for whom you want to have better health.

The recipients could be relatives, friends, team members, vendors, or someone you would like to make a discernable difference in their life. My goal is to make a positive impact on the lives of millions of people. To do that, I need your help.

I promise you overall it will be you who benefits the most. You're helping someone else find ideas to improve their eating habits and improve their overall health. You could alter the course of their life...possibly save someone's life. Because without you who gives it to them, they might never have found *Jaded Health Every Day Health Choices*.

Write down five people you will give a copy of this book to:

_____

_____

_____

_____

Thank you for doing this for me.
More than anything else, I wish you good HEALTH.
David Medansky

If what you have read, resonates with you –

I would love for you to leave an honest review on Amazon or Goodreads.

Hack Your Habits in 30 Minutes or Less Using The Kennedy Method©

By John Kennedy

"Never leave that til tomorrow that you can do now."
- Benjamin Franklin

In our daily lives, habits are the threads that weave our routines and guide our actions. From the moment we wake up to the time we lay our heads to rest, habits shape the contours of our existence. But what if we could mold these habits consciously? What if we could hack into the very fabric of our routines, redirecting the threads to create a masterpiece of personal development?

Welcome to "Hack Your Habits," a journey into the fascinating realm of habit transformation and the neuroscience that underlies it. This chapter is your guide to understanding, breaking, replacing, and creating habits that resonate with the life you desire to lead.

Steps to Hack Your Habits:

It's important to set aside about 30 minutes of uninterrupted time. However, it might take less. Plan for 30 minutes and celebrate if you finish early!

The easiest way to get started is by using a 3x5 card.

On the unlined side of the card, write the name of your new habit – something that signifies what you want to accomplish. Some examples include:

- Get up on time.
- Doing some sort of physical activity every day such as walking.
- Stop eating sweets.

Then on the same side of the card, describe your "Why" for the new habit, something meaningful to you such as,

- Feel stronger and more confident.
- Have time to get my day started without stress.
- Feel in control of my eating and be healthier.

Implementing The Kennedy Method

1. First, define the new habit (usually the non-lined side). Your objective is to transfer conscious processing to the unconscious known as Zombie System. Zombie System is the term neuroscientists use for the transfer of mental processing from the conscious to the unconscious to form a habit. A habit is a Zombie System because it is done without thought or thinking about it.

Next, **break your new habit that you want to create into steps (five steps is a good number to attempt)** and write them on the other side (usually the lined side) of the card. Too few and it won't make a meaningful change, more than five and it can get hard to implement. Simple and efficient is best.

The first step should be the trigger you have identified to initiate the habit.

Once you've defined your new habit in terms of steps, visualize yourself performing the steps. Be aware of any tension you might feel – that's a sign that you might be missing a detail. For example, if your new habit includes brushing your teeth and you write down, 'Pick up a toothbrush and start brushing,' you might have missed adding the toothpaste.

Once you can think yourself through the process comfortably, it's time to incorporate the second part of The Kennedy Method known as *Robust Stimulation*. Robust Stimulation is defined as stimulating the parts of the brain critical to executive function while simultaneously stimulating the brain's connections to the real world.

2. Physically go to where you will use your new habit and perform your new habit, step by step, engaging all parts of your brain and body that you will use. Then take a minute to think through what you have just done and repeat it. Again. And again. And again. Wash, rinse and repeat are the secret. Every time you repeat the process the same way, using all the brain/body connections in harmony, the stronger the connections and the faster you create a new habit. Once you start the process, you may notice after a few repetitions that you begin to anticipate the trigger, which releases dopamine and gives you that feeling of excitement. Now, you will find that you are beginning to complete it without thinking.

3. Now you can apply the same process to create or modify another habit. Using what you've learned will make the process even faster the next time – that's the Agile approach. The Agile approach is defined as utilizing a cycle of continuous improvement.

The following are several examples of completely different habits formed using this process, from real people.

GETTING OUT OF BED ON TIME

When asked, most people admit that when the alarm goes off, they hit the snooze button. Some even prepare for this by setting their alarm early or use a second alarm. They then proceed to repeat this several times before they finally jump out of bed in a panic and rush through their morning to get to where they need to go on time, often flustered, and stressed.

The folks that do this have unknowingly created a "hit the snooze button" habit." The more they do this, no matter how determined they are to get up on time, they make it easier to fail.

Here's what to do to hack the snooze button habit.

On a non-pressure day, perhaps a Saturday afternoon when you have some free time, on a 3 x 5 card write on the non-lined side:

> **Name it** – Get out of bed on time.
> **Why?** To start my day in control, without stress.

On the lined side write:

---

1. When the alarm goes off, get out of bed.
2. Turn off the alarm.
3. Make the bed – remembering Admiral McCraven's advice, start your day with an accomplishment by making your bed.
4. Start to walk away.
5. Turn around, look at your bed and say, "Good job, it's going to be a great day!"

Now use The Kennedy Method to implement the new habit in 5 steps:

RINSE AND REPEAT

Set your alarm to wake up in two minutes. Get back into bed, pull the covers up. Read, out loud, the steps on your card. Wait for the alarm to go off, do the steps quickly.

1. When the alarm goes off, get out of bed.
2. Turn off the alarm.
3. Make the bed – Remembering Admiral McCraven's advice, start your day with an accomplishment by making your bed.
4. Start to walk away.
5. Turn around, look at your made bed and say, "Good job, it's going to be a great day!"

Repeat this several more times. You will find that after a few repetitions, you will be completely relaxed and primed to do your new habit. The anticipation will release dopamine, reinforcing the good feeling you will have when you accomplish your new habit. You will quickly find that you will do it without thinking and feel good about it. When that happens, you are ready for Monday morning! You will go to bed the night before excited to wake up with the alarm and get your day started right.

Let's try a different habit. This is one we worked through at a conference when I invited the audience to suggest habits they wanted to change or create.

WORKOUT WHEN GETTING HOME FROM WORK

This was from a man who was determined to get healthy for his family as well as himself. He was committed to working out when he got home from work but found that once he walked in the door and saw his wife and family, he felt guilty leaving and was using that as an excuse.

This is how he hacked his habit.

On a non-pressure day, in his case, a Saturday afternoon when he had some free time, he did the following:

On a 3 x 5 card he wrote,

Named it – Workout after work.
Why? – Be healthier for himself and for his family as he gets older. In this case it's important to explain to his family that he's doing it for them.

Next he defined the new habit in 5 steps on the Lined Side of the Note Card:

---

1. The night before he puts his gym bag by the door.
2. When he gets home from work, he drops his work things by the door.
3. He gives his wife a kiss and tells her he loves her and that he is going to work out.
4. He picks up his workout bag.
5. He goes to the car and gets inside.

Do steps 1 through 5.

1. Place the gym bag by the door and step outside (even sit in your car)
2. Open the front door and drop your work things by the door.
3. Give your wife a kiss and tell you love her and that you are going to work out.
4. Pick up your workout bag.
5. Physically leave and go to your car.

Say to yourself, "That was a great workout!"

Repeat steps 1 through 5.

Not only did he create the working out after work habit he wanted, he also made his wife happy by kissing her and telling her that he loved her ten times in less than 30 minutes!

Once you define the trigger, a motive and the desired result, you can hack any habit, even in sports.

One of my clients was an amateur tennis player and over the short time we worked together his ranking rose from 2.5 to 4.5. One of his issues was difficulty looking at his racquet instead of down court when the ball hit it. He pointed out that the best players in the world always watched the ball hit their racquet, and as much as he tried to remember, he couldn't do it consistently.

So, The Kennedy Method to the rescue!

I told him to write down why this was important to him - to win more matches, less frustration after games, etc. **And the trigger-the ball hitting his racquet.** I then told him to go to the court by the backboard on a day when he had some quiet time. He had been instructed to hit the ball against the backboard repeatedly and force himself to look at it as it hit his racquet, using the same swings he uses when he plays.

As he got better, he could move back for a full swing and up close for volleys, both forehand and backhand.

Remember the **Kennedy Method** - conscious to unconscious execution, using all parts of the body used in the real action. After 30 minutes he had trained himself to look at the ball hitting the racquet without thinking about it. Something he was now able to do consistently in matches unconsciously, freeing his brain to strategize on placement, etc.

HABIT HIJACKING

Habit Hijacking is not habit stacking. Habit stacking is adding a new desirable habit to one you already rely on. Habit hijacking is changing a bad habit by inserting a short new habit in front of the habit that you want to change.

It starts with the same trigger as the bad habit. However, by inserting the good habit into the habit loop before the process starts, it can radically change the outcome.

For example, immediately looking at your device when a message notification is received is a bad habit. Texting while driving can be very dangerous especially for younger people who:

1) are not experienced drivers, and

2) have developed FOMO (Fear of missing out) dependence and answering messages immediately.

My cell carrier has a big message that appears whenever I go to pay my bill that says "Take the Pledge! Don't text and drive!". However, as previously observed, telling yourself to get up on time and not hit the "snooze button" the next morning will not create the habit that you need to do it.

Just like the "snooze button" habit you were creating, when you look at your phone hundreds of times during the day, you are creating a "look at my phone" habit that is very hard to break because of the repetition you have done up until this point in time.

It's not only young people who have this issue. One of my clients had just launched a website and was anxious to get the notifications that people had visited it. So, she also struggled with the same FOMO "look at my phone" bad habit.

The solution to both instances is to insert a 10 second count between the trigger – the notification – and the process that starts the bad habit – looking at the phone.

Here's how to do it. First, identify your why. For instance, it could save your life, avoid being rude during conversations, or losing focus during calls, webinars, etc.

Ten seconds is not that long a time for the person messaging you to wait, in fact it probably happens naturally, and no one notices.

So, the new insertion habit is to count to 10 after the notification and before looking at your phone. And, just like the habits you created earlier, we'll use the Kennedy method to make it a new habit very quickly.

As described earlier, use your 3 x 5 card and write down the reason to create the ten second count and the benefits (listed above) then the steps:

The "Trigger" is your phone alert notifying you of a text message or email. To begin, find a quiet time without distractions. Set your alert (you can use a timer) for 30 seconds. When it goes off, count to 10 before deliberately looking at your phone.

Next, put your phone back and reset the alert timer for 30 seconds. After several times, set the timer for 1 minute - this will extend the in between time and the anticipation space. Finally set the timer for 5 minutes and follow the process when it goes off - count to 10 then look at your phone.

You have just created a conscious space to evaluate whether to look at your phone or not before you do. If this happens while driving, you now have a chance to say to yourself "Maybe I should pullover before I look", or during time with other people "maybe I should continue this conversation with my friend and look later." From now on you have taken control and given yourself a choice to evaluate your actions.

With these two powerful Kennedy Method "habit hacking" techniques you can use to literally change or create any habit in less than 30 minutes!

For more information on how to experience the most powerful Peak Performance program, visit the www.hackyourhabitsin30.com where you will find some tools to help you.

Bio:

John Kennedy, Neuroplastician, is the Director for the Mental Performance Institute and premier Executive Brain Coach. John is also a number one International Bestselling Author. He developed his innovative Combat Brain Training method at the request of the US Marine Corps in 2007. He has successfully helped thousands of people and teams dramatically improve their lives by quickly improving their mental ability regardless of starting performance baseline. You can contact John Kennedy at:

The Kennedy Method™
847-791-1825
john@combatbraintraining.com
www.mentalperformanceinstitute.org

The Last House

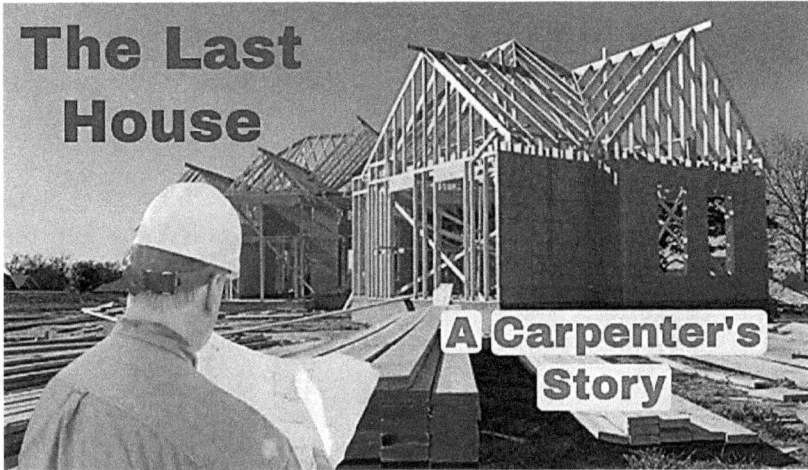

One afternoon, a carpenter, who had been with the same company for more than 30 years, told his boss that he was ready to end his career and spend time with his wife and family. He would miss his work, however, he felt he needed to spend more time with the people who were important to him.

The owner of the company was saddened by this news, because this carpenter had been a good, dependable employee for many years. He asked the carpenter if he could do him a favor and build just one more house.

Reluctantly, and after a bit of persuasion from the owner, the carpenter agreed to build just one more home.

The carpenter's heart just wasn't in building this last home. He lost focus and dreamed of spending time with his family. Because he was not fully engaged in this project, his normal work ethic waned, and his efforts were mediocre at best. He chose to use inexpensive and inferior materials. He cut corners wherever he could. The quality was shoddy. It was a poor way to finish such a dedicated career that he once had.

When the carpenter had finished, his boss came to inspect the house. He gave the key to the carpenter and said, "This house is my gift to you for all the hard work you have done for me over the years."

The carpenter was surprised and overwhelmed with his boss' generosity. He graciously accepted the gift. After his boss left, the carpenter sat for a moment to ponder his decision to put forth less than his best effort. Had he known the home was for him and his family, he would have made his usual effort to create a high-quality home.

The same idea applies to how you take care of your own body. Dr. Bob Martin, Certified Clinical Nutritionist (C.C.N.), host of "The Dr. Bob Martin Show," the largest syndicated alternative health show in the U.S., said, "If you wear out your body, where are you going to live?"

Each and every day that you wake up you have an opportunity to do your best and be your best. Yet many of you often do mediocre work. Why? Shouldn't we strive to improve each day?

As we get older, we find ourselves shocked that our lives aren't what we had hoped they would be. The "house" (our bodies) we built to live in has a lot of flaws due to a lack of effort. Unfortunately, you are unable to go back and rebuild it in a day or two. It takes time to repair the damage done. There is a saying, "Life is a do-it-yourself project." And so is maintaining and taking care of your body. Your attitude and daily food choices help build the quality of life you will have in the future. Build carefully.

"Living a healthy life is a struggle because of the messages being propounded upon you every day."

- David Medansky,
The Health Guy

What Others Are Saying

"David Medansky offers an achievable, realistic, and simple approach for healthy and permanent weight loss that anyone can do."
—**Jack Canfield**, New York Times best-selling coauthor of *Chicken Soup for the Soul®*

"David Medansky has been where you are, he's been where all of us have been… he lost 50 pounds in four months. So, he can probably assist you with your weight-loss journey… David is a good guy. I know him personally."
—**Dean Cain**, Superman, *Lois & Clark*

"If you have tried every diet or weight-loss program without being able to keep the weight off, David brilliantly distills simple changes to your daily eating habits and routines to shed your weight and keep it off."
—**Hal Elrod**, best-selling author of *The Miracle Morning and The Miracle Equation*

"David Medansky does a masterful job of exposing many of today's diet weight loss myths."
—**Kyle Wilson**, author of *Success Habits of Super Achievers* and Founder, Jim Rohn International and KyleWilson.com

"If you're ready to take your life and business to better levels and sustain continuous growth and improvement, then you must work with my friend David. Here's the great thing – he focuses on getting you laser-focused, cutting you through all of the clutter and inspiring you to produce outcomes!

He's on a mission through his speaking, live events, coaching and online publications to make a HUGE positive difference in the lives of as many people as possible. And he comes from the heart and genuinely wants to help others. Do yourself a favor and work with David today! You'll be so grateful you did!"

—**James Malinchak**, Featured on ABCs hit TV show, *Secret Millionaire*, best-selling author of 20 books, delivered 3,000+ presentations and 1,000+ consultations

I think about David Medansky losing 50 pounds and how it gave him the passion to help other people to lose weight. David helps you overcome the weight-loss challenges you will face by showing you how you can eat within the guidelines of what you are already doing.

—**Kevin Harrington,** The Original Shark on the hit TV show, *Shark Tank*, and responsible for more than $5 billion in sales.

When David Medansky asked me to write the foreword to his book *If Not Now, When?* I was honored and eager to share my message about his work, as he has been a significant part of changing the world's weight mindset in a healthy manner. I think of David as a true innovator and crusader for people's health.

—**Lori Shemek Ph.D., CNC**, best-selling author of *Fire-Up Your Fat Burn!* and *How to Fight FATflammation!*

David Medansky sets forth scientifically proven, practical, everyday principles to successfully reduce weight and keep it off.

—**Dr. David Friedman, N.D., D.C.**, best-selling award-winning author of *Food Sanity*

If you've been neglecting your health, David Medansky provides a simple yet powerful solution to start living a healthy life and improving your health.

—**Robyn Chubinsky**, L.Ac, MSOM, Dipl. Ac, Fire Horse Integrated Wellness PLC

About David

David Medansky was born and raised in Chicago and now resides in Phoenix with his beautiful wife Debra.

He graduated with a bachelor's degree from the University of South Florida and has a Juris Doctorate from the University of Arizona Law School.

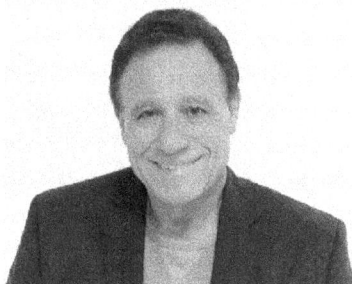

David practiced law for thirteen years until 2005 when he left law for health issues. David is an international best-selling author of *Stop Dieting Start Thinning, Discover Your Thinner Self, If Not Now When? Break the Chains of Dieting and many more.*

At age 61, David was obese and told by his doctor that he had a 95 percent chance of a fatal heart attack. David's doctor told him to find a new doctor because he did not believe David could lose weight and he did not want him dying on his watch. That was the pivotal point, where David realized the severity of his condition and decided to find a way to lose weight and keep it off. During the next four months David was able to shed 50 pounds, which was 25 percent of his total body weight.

David spent his law career seeing both sides of the fence. Honest people and dishonest people. And during his weight loss journey he realized that when it comes to the food and weight-loss industries, sadly there are more dishonest people than there are those telling the truth. That's what makes losing weight so difficult. David learned 9 Simple Golden Rules to live a healthy life and is on a mission to share this message with the world.

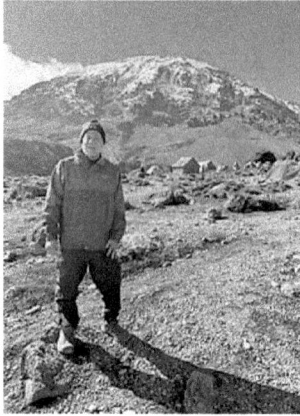

In June 2022, at age 67, David hiked Mt. Kilimanjaro. Kilimanjaro, at 5,895 meters (19,341 feet), is the highest single free-standing mountain above sea level in the world. It is the fourth highest mountain in the world. It is referred to as the "Roof Top of Africa."

www.ingramcontent.com/pod-product-compliance
Lightning Source LLC
Chambersburg PA
CBHW052128270326
41930CB00012B/2805